Okay . . . I've Gone Through Weight Loss Surgery, Now What Do I Do?!

Okay . . . I've Gone Through Weight Loss Surgery, Now What Do I Do?!

Joanne M. Moff PA-C

To order additional copies of this book, contact:
Xlibris Corporation
1-888-795-4274
www.Xlibris.com
Orders@Xlibris.com
60279

Contents

Dedication

This book is dedicated to all of you who, after years of struggling with your weight, have chosen to take a very big step toward becoming healthier. You braved the world of bariatric surgery. While it may feel like you're alone in your journey to better health, you're not. Your family, friends, coworkers, health care providers, and other bariatric patients want to see you succeed; and we're here to help you succeed. So hold your head up high and start living your new life!

Disclaimer

The medical information provided in this book is meant to help you better understand the physical changes your body is going through as a result of your bariatric surgery. You will not see every possible change mentioned. Nor will you see every possible complication or problem that can result from your surgery.

Brand names that are used are intended to offer you suggestions on specific products that are available in stores and on the Internet. These products are by no means the only products available to you.

If you have any questions or concerns that are not addressed in this book, please contact your doctor, physician assistant, nurse, or other health care provider. If the information given by your health care provider conflicts with information given in this book, follow the guidance of your health care provider.

Acknowledgments

Rita M. Anderson, MD, PhD, FACS, specializes in bariatric surgery. She is the medical director of New Life Weight Loss Surgery Center, a center of excellence by the American Society for Metabolic and Bariatric Surgeons (ASMBS). New Life Weight Loss Surgery Center is located in the Physicians Office Building adjacent to the Kettering Medical Center in Kettering, Ohio.

Thank you for listening and being receptive to my ideas, supporting my work and pushing me to strive for more.

New Life Weight Loss Surgery Center Team
Thank you for allowing me to bounce ideas off you as well as sharing ways through which we can help our patients succeed.

David P. Evans, PA-C, has been a practicing physician assistant for twenty-eight years. He has experience in both general and cardiothoracic surgery. He recently changed his focus to bariatric surgery and works with Dr. Rita Anderson at the Kettering Medical Center.

Thank you for engaging in countless and lengthy conversations and watching as my brain "stormed" with ideas.

My family, both immediate and extended, most especially my parents, who are together with each other in heaven, and my six sisters, scattered far and wide, *thank you for your excitement, motivation, and support.*

Introduction

You made the decision to undergo weight loss surgery—**Lap Band**, **Roux-en-Y**, or **Biliopancreatic Diversion with/without Duodenal Switch** (BPD)—and it may have taken you years to get to this point. And now you've had your surgery. What happens next is up to you. You've been provided with a very powerful tool—whether it's the Lap Band, Roux-en-Y, or BPD—to help you with your weight loss goals. But how will you make sure you use your tool fully? How can you make sure you are doing what you need to do to maintain your new lifestyle?

To help keep you on track early after surgery as well as years on down the road, it is important to find support in others who have gone through the same thing. That's what this book is all about—offering you support. Some of the information in this book is taken from medical books, journals, and various Web sites. But some of the suggestions are from other patients—patients who have undergone weight loss surgery and know what you are going through. You have an opportunity to read other patients' suggestions and words of advice.

Before your surgery, you were probably told that life afterward would be different, especially with regard to eating and drinking. You were given lots of handouts with information. You went through classes on diet, nutrition, and exercise. As you listened to the instruction, you may have thought, *This is no big deal. It's easy! I can do this.*

Right after your surgery, you may feel like your brain is being overloaded. You're hearing AGAIN how and what you can eat, which you're told will take time and lots of trial and error. For the first few days after your surgery, your mind may be fuzzy, between the effects of the anesthetic medications that were given to you during surgery and the pain medications you're taking after your surgery. You may not be comprehending instructions your doctor and nurse are giving you. You may even start to feel panic. You have to actually DO what you were taught to do. Suddenly it's not so easy to sip fluids all day long or eat your food slowly. Take a deep breath and relax. Remember all those handouts and education classes? Use that information to help you. Use this support book to teach you and guide you in your new lifestyle too. You CAN do this.

Are you wondering if it even matters if you follow all those crazy new ways of eating and drinking? Sure it does. Think of your body as a car. Remember when you got your first car? There was a lot to learn about how to take care of it and keep it working properly. If you didn't take care of your car the way the manufacturer recommended, your car would not run properly, and you wouldn't get two hundred thousand miles out of it. It's the same with your surgery. You need to follow your surgeon's recommendations to "overhaul" your body and improve your "mileage." Your surgery is the engine, the main thing driving your weight loss. The water you drink is like the oil in your car. Your car will not run smoothly, and the engine will seize up without oil. The proteins and other foods you eat are the gasoline. You need to fill the tank with good-quality fuel periodically to keep the car running. The vitamins and minerals you take are like the antifreeze, transmission fluid, brake fluid, and power steering fluid your car needs to keep each part of the car functioning properly and running well as a whole. Your body needs exercise like your car needs to be driven to keep all systems running more efficiently and effectively. You want to get "two hundred thousand miles" out of your surgery?

As you read this support book, you will find that each chapter tackles a specific problem: drinking enough liquids, eating enough protein, taking the proper vitamins, getting exercise, dealing with depression, finding different meal ideas, dealing with problems and complications, and moving forward after your surgery. You are reminded of the lifestyle changes you need to make. But more than that, the reasons behind the lifestyle changes are explained. And you are given specific examples of how to make those changes real in your life.

Your surgery is the powerful tool you chose to get you started on the road to better health. But like the engine of your car, your tool can only take you so far. It is up to you to keep all the parts of your "car" working properly. This is your new life and your new lifestyle. Your journey toward better health has begun. Let this support book help you continue along the journey, from the first day after your surgery and every day thereafter.

FLUIDS AND DRINKING HABITS

DRINKING SIXTY-FOUR OUNCES OF FLUID EVERY DAY?

Water . . . water . . . water! You're going to hear a lot about water. Why do we make such a big deal about water? Why is it so important to drink? Well, there are a lot of reasons why.

First of all, your body is made up of about 60 percent water, which helps to maintain the balance of fluids in your body. What fluids? Fluids used in blood pressure, circulation, digestion, heart rate, transportation and absorption of nutrients, saliva, and temperature regulation. Your body is constantly losing fluid through such things as urine, stool, breathing, and sweat. When you have periods of diarrhea, fevers, excessive sweating, frequent urination, or vomiting, your body is losing even more fluid. So it is necessary to replenish what you lose. You know that feeling of thirst that you get? That's your brain telling you, "Water . . . I need water!"

Second, water helps out your kidneys. Your kidneys have a very important job: cleansing your body of pollution. As long as you get enough water, your kidneys can efficiently get rid of toxins floating around in your body. While you are losing weight, your body has more toxins and waste to get rid of, and water helps to flush out all that waste. You've probably noticed your urine take on different colors (admit it—you've looked). The lighter it is, the better hydrated you are and the better your kidneys are working to get rid of toxins. The darker it is, the more dehydrated you may be and the more concentrated the toxins coming out of you. When you don't drink enough water, your body goes into panic mode and starts storing it throughout your body, instead of getting rid of it. And it stores it in weird places like your hands, wrists, belly, legs, ankles, and feet. Moral of the story—drink up! It sounds crazy, but drinking more water will actually help you get rid of extra water.

Another reason why water is so important: metabolism of fat. Here's what happens. In order to help your body function, your liver takes stored fat and converts it into energy. How does it do this? Your body, your liver, needs water to flush toxins from the stored fat cells. This helps the liver to metabolize the stored fat. But the fat cells also have to be free of extra water. When you're dehydrated, your body is in panic mode and is retaining water. This means that the fat cells are holding on to extra water, therefore, making it harder for the liver to metabolize the stored fat.

The liver also has the important job of helping out the kidneys. Remember, your kidneys have the vital responsibility of filtering your blood of toxins and sending them out of your body. When your kidneys aren't working as well—which occurs when you don't drink enough water—the liver steps in to bail out the kidneys. This causes the liver to focus more on holding on to fluid instead of burning fat, which means that your body and fat cells are holding on to excess water. So if the liver is helping out the kidneys, it can't work on metabolizing fat as efficiently. When this happens, the liver stores fat instead of converting it into energy. When you're trying to lose weight, you don't want to be storing fat. So you need to be drinking plenty of water to keep your kidneys happy and your liver occupied with more important things—burning fat!

When you first start to increase the amount of water you drink, be prepared; you will be making a lot of trips to the bathroom. But this won't last forever. What's happening is your body is flushing the water it has been storing over all those years of being in survival mode. Keep the faith and keep drinking water. As your body realizes it is getting the water it needs, it will begin to get rid of what it doesn't need. In fact, your body will begin getting rid of water in your ankles, hips, thighs, and maybe even around your belly that it has been storing in case of emergency. Your body will no longer be in survival mode and will no longer need to store the water. Eventually the frequent trips to the bathroom will slow down too.

If you drink coffee or tea (including iced tea) to get some of your fluids, be cautious as you may actually be hurting yourself. You probably know coffee and tea contain caffeine, and caffeine is a diuretic. Diuretics make you, you guessed it, pee like a "you-know-what." So you're really not helping yourself by drinking caffeine. Caffeine can do other bad things too like cause ulcers, damage the lining of your stomach, play a part in calcium loss, raise your blood pressure, and raise your heart rate. Decaffeinated coffee and tea are okay.

Alcoholic beverages are another fluid of which to be cautious. They really shouldn't count toward your fluids and are actually something you should try to avoid. First of all, alcohol is high in calories—empty calories. You need to make sure your calories count now more than ever. Second, alcohol is absorbed more quickly by your body, making you intoxicated from drinking very small amounts.

Water is important for yet another reason. It flushes out impurities from your skin, giving you a naturally clean and glowing complexion. It also makes your skin look younger and less wrinkled. Who doesn't want younger, more glowing skin? Skin that is dehydrated looks and feels dry. Your skin may also become saggy as you lose weight. Water may plump up those skin cells when they are hydrated properly. (Exercise will also help with preventing sagging skin, especially resistance exercises that build muscle.) Water also improves muscle tone. Muscles that have all the water they need contract more easily, which is important as you start exercising. You will be helping to make your workouts more effective by drinking water. So be sure to "knock back" some water before, during, and after exercising. Also remember that as you exercise, you will sweat—yet another reason to drink water.

That brings us to another problem: thirst. Don't let yourself get thirsty. If you feel thirsty, you're already becoming dehydrated. Drink, drink, drink. Don't worry too much about drowning. Your body—your kidneys—knows what to do with the flood of water coming its way.

Drinking isn't the only way you can get water. Did you know that many foods you eat contain water like fruits, vegetables, and meat? Well, they do. Some high-protein foods contain lots of water, including eggs and fish, which are roughly 70 percent water. Most fruits and vegetables contain between 80 percent and 90 percent water. The following are examples of foods with high water content and the percentage of water they contain:

Apple	84%
Broccoli	91%
Carrot	87%
Grapefruit	91%
Lettuce	95%
Milk	89%
Oranges	90%
Watermelon	92%
Yogurt	85%

About 20 percent of the water you get comes from the foods you eat. In fact, food with high water content (especially fruits and vegetables) is higher in volume, requires more chewing, is absorbed more slowly by your body, and makes you feel fuller longer. After your surgery, though, fruits, vegetables and meat aren't the kinds of foods you will be eating right away. So you will not be "eating" the same amount of fluid as you were before your surgery. How are you going to get the fluid you're missing? By drinking it. Even after you begin eating meat, vegetables, and fruits again, you will be consuming much less than you did before you had surgery; so you will still be "eating" less water in your diet. What does this mean? Drink up!

Are you getting the hint that water is very important? Now you need to decide how you are going to get it. How do you like your water? Fresh from the tap? If you have hard water or well water, this may not be your first choice. You can reduce lead and other contaminants in your water and retain fluoride by using water filters, either faucet mounted (PŪR or Brita) or pitchers (PŪR or Brita). If your refrigerator has a water dispenser, you can also get a filter for this (Brita). If this sounds like too much trouble, there is also bottled water (which is basically filtered tap water).

If drinking plain water turns you off, try flavored water. Many varieties contain electrolytes and vitamins. Just be sure to watch out for those containing sugar as this may cause dumping syndrome, especially in Roux-en-Y patients.

Sugar also contains calories, and when you're trying to lose weight, every calorie counts. Here are a number of examples of flavored waters that you can find in your local grocery stores and on the Internet:

Aquafina
- ☺ Alive—contains vitamins, antioxidants, and Splenda
- ☺ Flavor Splash—contains natural flavors and Splenda
- ☺ Sparkling—carbonated water containing natural fruit flavors and Aspartame

Dasani
- ☺ Plus—contains vitamins and natural fruit flavors
- ☺ Flavored water—contains natural flavors and Splenda

Fruit$_2$O
- ☺ Contains natural flavor and Splenda
- ☺ Vitamin-enhanced water—contains natural flavors

Glacéau
- ☺ Vitamin water
- ☺ Fruit water—contains electrolytes, no artificial sweeteners
- ☺ Smart water—contains electrolytes
- ☺ Vitamin energy—contains vitamins and natural caffeine

Hint
- ☺   Water with a hint of natural flavor
- ☺   No sugar or artificial sweeteners added
- ☺   Found in specialty markets, spas, and hotels
- ☺   More expensive (twenty-four sixteen-ounce bottles—$44)

Kellogg's Special K Protein Water—contains five grams of protein, sugar, and Splenda

Ocean Spray flavor packets
- ☺   Five calories per serving
- ☺   Contain Aspartame

PŪR
- ☺   Flavor cartridges can be added to filtered water

If you have trouble tolerating artificial sweeteners and choose to use sugar, try Kool-Aid singles. They have only seven grams of sugar per packet. Even diluted in sixty-four ounces of water, they are still flavorful.

Drinking plain water and flavored water may still have some of you wanting more. Either you want more flavor or are worried about becoming deficient in your electrolytes, so you decide to drink sports drinks. The major problem with this type of fluid is the amount of sugar per serving. Again, calories are a concern as well as the possibility of causing dumping syndrome. So read the nutrition labels carefully. The following are some of the more popular sports drinks and their sugar content:

All Sport
☺   Sixteen grams of sugar per eight-ounce serving

Gatorade
☺   Thirteen grams of sugar per eight-ounce serving
☺   Contains the electrolytes sodium and potassium

G2 (Gatorade 2)
☺   Seven grams of sugar per eight-ounce serving
☺   Contains the electrolytes sodium and potassium

PowerAde
☺   Fifteen grams of sugar per eight ounce serving
☺   Contains the electrolytes sodium and potassium

Propel
☺   Two grams of sugar per eight-ounce serving

Are you beginning to appreciate how important it is to get your fluids in every day? Do you still feel overwhelmed at the thought of drinking sixty-four ounces? Here are some suggestions that you can try to help you get all that liquid in every day:

☺ Keep a water bottle with you at all times.

☺ Try drinking protein shakes—this can count for both your fluid and protein intake.

☺ Drink cold water—according to some studies, cold water is absorbed more quickly by your stomach.

☺ Remember, if drinking plain water is not palatable to you, flavored water or low-calorie drinks are okay.

☺ Don't drink liquids within at least thirty minutes of your meals (before and after).

You've taken the hint, and you're drinking as much as you can. Unfortunately, you may develop a pressure feeling in your chest or even the hiccups. Why did this happen, and what do you do about it?

You may be swallowing air when you drink. One way to prevent this is by avoiding the use of straws. "What difference does it make if I use a straw?" you ask. Well, let's think about that. When you put a straw into your glass, there will be fluid in the straw but only up to the level of the fluid in the glass. What's above the fluid level? Air. When you start to drink from the straw, the first thing you get is air, and then you get the fluid. With your stomach pouch as small as it is, it doesn't take much to fill it up. The last thing you want to do is fill it up with air because too much can actually cause you discomfort.

Another way to prevent hiccups and a pressure feeling in your chest is to avoid drinking carbonated drinks. Similar idea as with the straw, when you drink carbonated drinks, you're filling your small stomach pouch with air. However, if you desperately need your Mountain Dew, you can still drink it. Just be sure to add lots of ice and stir your drink with a metal utensil. This will decrease the carbonation and help prevent those uncomfortable side effects.

And finally, drink slowly. Do not gulp your liquids. You're probably used to drinking fast, and now you have to really concentrate on taking your time. Filling your stomach pouch slowly will help prevent pain, pressure, and hiccups.

All right! Now that you're drinking plenty of water and other fluids, let's move on to protein.

PROTEIN AND EATING HABITS

CONSUMING FIFTY TO ONE HUNDRED GRAMS OF PROTEIN EVERY DAY?

Protein . . . protein . . . protein! Now we focus on the ever-important protein. Why do we give so much attention to protein? Well, let me tell you. Protein is found all throughout your body, in your muscles (bet you already guessed that), your bones, your skin, your hair (you may have guessed that one too), and virtually every other part of your body. Proteins make up the enzymes that power chemical reactions in your body—yes, you are a living chemistry lab—and the hemoglobin that carries oxygen in your blood. Amino acids are the building blocks of proteins; think of them as Legos that when snapped together build something more useful. But your body doesn't store these. You have to get amino acids and, therefore proteins, every day from the foods you eat.

But not all food sources of protein are created equally. Face it—that big, juicy, flame-broiled steak will give you a whopping serving of protein; but along with it will come a lot of saturated fat! You can do better for yourself by eating poultry or fish, which are the best animal sources of protein. You feel like a nut? Nuts are a great source of protein too. Just watch the saturated fat content in those too. You know how your mom always told you to eat your vegetables? Well these can also give you good sources of protein. So eat your beans and whole grains.

Following your surgery, you're eating a lot less, and you're losing weight quickly. Your body begins to use your muscles—a.k.a. protein—to help meet its energy requirements. If you get enough protein in your diet, your body goes after that first for energy. But if you don't get enough protein in your diet, you can have problems with loss of your muscle mass. You could also develop problems with your body's immune system not working as well. Your heart and lungs may weaken too. What's the moral of the story? Eat protein!

Okay, so you have to get a lot of protein in every day for the rest of your life. If you underwent the Lap Band or Roux-en-Y surgeries, you need to get a minimum of fifty grams of protein in every day. If you underwent the BPD, you need to get a whopping 100 grams of protein in every day. Remember that these are minimum daily requirements. As you start to exercise and, especially if you do weight lifting or resistance training, you will need to get more protein in your diet to help build those muscles.

This sounds overwhelming, trying to take in so many grams of protein. But it is not as difficult as you may think. You can make or buy shakes that contain anywhere from thirty to fifty grams of protein. Do you have a blender? Do you like frozen shakes? Then skip over to chapter 7 "Recipes." There you can find a recipe on how to make twenty-one different variations of one shake. There are also many foods you can eat that will provide higher grams of protein per serving. Not sure where to find all these good sources? Take a look at the following table that lists excellent sources of protein:

Food	Serving Size	Grams
Almonds	¼ cup	7.0
Beef sirloin, grilled	3 ounces	26.0
Chicken salad	½ cup	18.0
Chicken, roasted dark meat	3 ounces	22.0
Chicken, roasted white meat	3 ounces	26.0
Cottage cheese 2 percent	½ cup	16.0
Egg, large	1	7.0
Ground beef, lean, grilled	3 ounces	22.0
Halibut, broiled	3 ounces	23.0
Ham, sliced deli	2 ounces	14.5
Milk 2 percent	½ cup	4.0
Mozzarella cheese	1 ounce	8.0
Peanut butter	2 tablespoons	8.5
Provolone cheese	1 ounce	7.0
Red snapper, broiled	3 ounces	22.0
Ricotta cheese, part skim	½ cup	14.0
Scallops, broiled	3 ounces	18.0
Shrimp, steamed	3 ounces	21.0
Sole, broiled	3 ounces	21.0
Tuna, grilled	3 ounces	23.0
Tuna, water-packed	3 ounces	22.0
Turkey, roasted dark meat	3 ounces	24.0
Turkey, roasted white meat	3 ounces	25.0
Turkey, sliced deli	2 ounces	13.0
Yogurt, low fat	½ cup	6.5

If you choose to eat protein bars, try to find those that contain twenty to thirty-five grams of protein and two to eight net impact carbohydrates. What are net impact carbohydrates (or carbs)? To compute this number, use the following equation:

$$\text{Net impact carbs} = \text{Total carbs} - \text{Dietary fiber} - \text{Sugar alcohols and other low glycemic carbs}$$

You want to watch the number of carbohydrates you get because when you're trying to lose weight, you really don't want to be eating that many. If you're trying to become the next greatest bodybuilder, then carbohydrates are what you want (along with all the protein). You also should be aware of the type of carbohydrates you are eating. There are two types: complex carbohydrates and simple carbohydrates. Complex carbohydrates generally take longer to digest and will therefore make you feel fuller longer. They usually contain fiber, vitamins, and minerals. Good examples of complex carbohydrates include vegetables, breads, cereals, legumes, and pasta. Simple carbohydrates are digested more quickly and will therefore empty from your stomach more quickly. Many usually contain refined sugars and only a few vitamins and minerals. Examples of simple carbohydrates include fruits, fruit juices, milk, yogurt, honey, molasses, maple syrup, and sugar. Avoiding simple carbohydrates is not necessary, but you do need to limit them. Just be aware that because you can only eat very small portions of food, you need to make everything you eat count.

Need some other even more specific ideas for getting protein in your diet? Try the following protein powders or protein drinks to meet your nutritional requirements:

Beneprotein
- ☺ High-quality whey protein powder
- ☺ Contains six grams of protein per serving
- ☺ Can be mixed with fluids and food

Optisource High-Protein Drink
- ☺ Contains twelve grams of protein in each four-ounce serving
- ☺ Specially designed for bariatric surgery patients

Unjury for Weight loss Surgery
- ☺ Contains the highest-quality whey protein isolate
- ☺ Contains twenty grams of protein
- ☺ Five great-tasting flavors from which to choose including chocolate, vanilla, strawberry sorbet, chicken soup, and unflavored

☺   Can be added to Jell-o and pudding to make a high-protein snack

Zoic Nutrition Drink

☺   Contains twenty-one grams of an all-natural protein blend with high-quality amino acid content

☺   No sugar added and no high fructose corn syrup

☺   Contains no gluten

☺   99 percent fat free

☺   99 percent lactose free

☺   Contains twenty-six essential vitamins and minerals as well as fiber, iron, and calcium

☺   Certified by the American Heart Association

☺   Flavors include vanilla and chocolate (strawberry flavor coming soon)

☺   Can be found at Meijer, Kroger, and Medicine Shoppe

☺   Inexpensive—cost is $5.99 for a four-pack

Other specific ideas for getting protein in your diet include:

☺   Carnation Instant Breakfast—tastes like chocolate milk!

☺   Oh Yeah! protein shake contains thirty grams of protein (found at GNC)

☺   Special K protein water contains five grams of protein

☺   For a protein-packed pudding, mix ricotta cheese with sugar-free pudding and milk and beat well

☺　　Canned wild Alaskan salmon contains about three thirteen-gram servings of protein (found at Trader Joe's)

☺　　Oh Yeah! chocolate and caramel protein bar contains twenty-six grams of protein and tastes like a Snickers bar (watch the sugar content—eight grams of sugar and twelve net carbs; you may only be able to eat half or one-third of the bar at one time)

You may find yourself tempted to turn to some of the diet foods out on the market to get lower-calorie-and-higher-protein foods and drinks. While this is okay, be sure to read the nutrition labels. (Reading nutrition labels should become a habit.) Some foods or drinks contain higher amounts of sugar, which can cause dumping syndrome .as well as weight gain. If you're not already familiar with dumping syndrome, here are some of the symptoms associated with it:

☹　　Nausea

☹　　Bloating

☹　　Abdominal pain

☹　　Diarrhea

☹　　Lightheadedness

☹　　Diaphoresis (breaking out in a sweat)

☹　　Palpitations

South Beach and Slim Fast offer many diet foods from which to choose. Following is a condensed list of some of the South Beach Diet convenience foods as well as somewhat comprehensive and up-to-date lists of Slim Fast products—two of the more popular diet products you can find. Some are higher in protein than others, and some have higher sugar content than others. This and other information can be found at their Web sites.

South Beach Diet Bars and Snacks

Calories	100-220
Calories from fat	25-110
Total fat	2-13 grams
Saturated fat	2-4 grams
Cholesterol	0-5 mg
Sodium	0-360 mg
Total carbohydrates	8-26 grams
Dietary fiber	2-6 grams
Sugars	1-7 grams
Protein	3-19 grams
Vitamin A	0-50%
Vitamin C	0-100%
Calcium	0-20%
Iron	2-25%

There are other South Beach Diet convenience foods not listed. These include frozen pizzas, wraps, dressings, and cookies. Depending on the type of surgery you had, you may or may not be able to tolerate these foods due to the amount of doughy bread, carbohydrates, or sugar.

Slim Fast Optima Shakes (serving size 1 can)

Calories	180-190
Fat calories	50
Total fat	5-6 grams
Saturated fat	2-2.5 grams
Trans fat	0 grams
Polyunsaturated fat	0.5 grams
Monounsaturated fat	2.5-3.5 grams
Cholesterol	5 mg
Sodium	200 mg
Potassium	550-600 mg
Total carbohydrates	23-25 grams
Fiber	5 grams
Sugars	17-18 grams
Protein	10 grams

Slim Fast Optima Meal Bars (serving size 1 bar)

Calories	180-220
Fat calories	40-50
Total fat	4.5-6 grams
Saturated fat	2.5-4 grams
Trans fat	0 grams
Cholesterol	0-less than 5 mg
Sodium	75-360 mg
Potassium	70-400 mg
Total carbohydrates	29-35 grams
Fiber	1-3 grams
Sugars	13-17 grams

Sugar alcohol	0-12 grams
Protein	8 grams

Slim Fast Optima Snack Bars (serving size 1 bar)

Calories	120-140
Fat calories	30-50
Total fat	3.5-6 grams
Saturated fat	0.5-3 grams
Trans fat	0 grams
Polyunsaturated fat	1 gram
Monounsaturated fat	3.5 grams
Cholesterol	0-5 mg
Sodium	70-190 mg
Total carbohydrates	19-21 grams
Fiber	Less than 1-2 grams
Sugars	7-12 grams
Sugar alcohol	1-9 grams
Protein	1-2 grams

Slim Fast Optima Powders (serving size 1 scoop)

Calories	110
Fat calories	25-35
Total fat	3-4 grams
Saturated fat	0.5 grams
Trans fat	0 grams
Polyunsaturated fat	0.5 grams
Monounsaturated fat	2-3 grams
Cholesterol	Less than 5 mg

Sodium	120-140 mg
Potassium	160-260 mg
Total carbohydrates	18 grams
Fiber	4-5 grams
Sugars	6-12 grams
Protein	2 grams

Slim Fast High Protein Shakes (serving size 1 can)

Calories	190
Fat calories	45
Total fat	5 grams
Saturated fat	2 grams
Trans fat	0 grams
Polyunsaturated fat	1 grams
Monounsaturated fat	2 grams
Cholesterol	10 mg
Sodium	220 mg
Potassium	550-600 mg
Total carbohydrates	23-24 grams
Fiber	5 grams
Sugars	13 grams
Protein	15 grams

Slim Fast High Protein Meal Bars (serving size 1 bar)

Calories	190-200
Fat calories	50-60
Total fat	6-7 grams
Saturated fat	2.5-3 grams

Trans fat	0 grams
Cholesterol	0-less than 5 mg
Sodium	200 mg
Potassium	270-300 mg
Total carbohydrates	20-21 grams
Fiber	2-9 grams
Sugars	8-18 grams
Protein	15 grams

Slim Fast High Protein Snack Bars (serving size 1 bar)

Calories	100-110
Fat calories	30-35
Total fat	3.5 grams
Saturated fat	0.5-2 grams
Trans fat	0 grams
Cholesterol	0-less than 5 mg
Sodium	90-120 mg
Potassium	65-70 mg
Total carbohydrates	12-16 grams
Fiber	0 grams
Sugars	5-7 grams
Sugar alcohol	0-9 grams
Protein	5-6 grams

Slim Fast High Protein Powders (serving size 1 scoop)

Calories	110
Fat calories	30
Total fat	3.5 grams

Saturated fat	0.5 grams
Trans fat	0 grams
Polyunsaturated fat	0.5 grams
Monounsaturated fat	2-2.5 grams
Cholesterol	Less than 5 mg
Sodium	130-140 mg
Potassium	160-200 mg
Total carbohydrates	13 grams
Fiber	4 grams
Sugars	6 grams
Protein	7 grams

Slim Fast Lower Carb Shakes (serving size 1 can)

Calories	180-190
Fat calories	80
Total fat	9 grams
Saturated fat	1.5 grams
Trans fat	0 grams
Polyunsaturated fat	1.5 grams
Monounsaturated fat	6 grams
Cholesterol	15 mg
Sodium	220-260 mg
Potassium	550 mg
Total carbohydrates	4-6 grams
Fiber	2-4 grams
Sugars	1 gram
Sugar alcohol	0 grams
Other carbohydrates	1 gram
Protein	20 grams

Slim Fast Lower Carb Snack Bars (serving size 1 bar)

Calories	120
Fat calories	40-45
Total fat	4.5-5 grams
Saturated fat	2-3 grams
Trans fat	0 grams
Cholesterol	Less than 5 mg
Sodium	70-80 mg
Total carbohydrates	15-21 grams
Fiber	1-2 grams
Sugars	Less than 1 gram
Sugar alcohol	12-18 grams
Other carbohydrates	0-2 grams
Protein	1-6 grams

Slim Fast Easy-to-Digest Shakes (serving size 1 can)

Calories	180
Fat calories	45
Total fat	5 grams
Saturated fat	1 gram
Trans fat	0 grams
Polyunsaturated fat	1 gram
Monounsaturated fat	3 grams
Cholesterol	Less than 5 mg
Sodium	220-240 mg
Potassium	500-600 mg
Total carbohydrates	24-26 grams

Fiber	3 grams
Sugars	20-21 grams
Protein	10 grams

Slim Fast Original Shakes (serving size 1 can)

Calories	220
Fat calories	25
Total fat	2.5-3 grams
Saturated fat	0.5-1 grams
Trans fat	0 grams
Polyunsaturated fat	0.5 grams
Monounsaturated fat	1.5 grams
Cholesterol	5 mg
Sodium	220 mg
Potassium	600 mg
Total carbohydrates	40 grams
Fiber	5 grams
Sugars	34-35 grams
Protein	10 grams

Slim Fast Original Meal Bars (serving size 1 bar)

Calories	140-220
Fat calories	45-50
Total fat	5-6 grams
Saturated fat	2.5-3.5 grams
Trans fat	0 grams
Cholesterol	Less than 5-5 mg

Sodium	70-160 mg
Potassium	70-150 mg
Total carbohydrates	19-36 grams
Fiber	2 grams
Sugars	12-20 grams
Protein	5-8 grams

Other than just discussing protein—which you now know is VERY important to your diet—it's good to have an overall understanding of how to eat now that you've had your surgery. Keep in mind that the first time you try a food, you may have problems eating it, but eventually you should be able to tolerate that particular food without difficulty. Or you may find that the first few times you eat a particular food, you have no problems at all. Then the fourth time you eat it, you do have difficulty. Don't panic; this is normal. Wait a few days and try that problem food again. Here are some additional guidelines for you to follow with regard to your diet in general. If these recommendations are different from what your surgeon has given you, follow your surgeon's advice.

How to Eat Following the Lap Band

For the first two weeks following surgery, you will be on an all-liquid diet, which should be low fat and low sugar. You will be slowly drinking four to six ounces of liquid six times a day. Be sure to drink your liquid meals three hours apart. Drink water BETWEEN meals.

a gastric band
placed laparoscopically

For the third, fourth, fifth, and sixth weeks following surgery, you will be on a pureed diet, eating foods that are the consistency of applesauce. At this point, you can slowly eat 1 ½ ounces of pureed protein with one ounce of pureed carbohydrate (preferably vegetables) six times a day. These meals should be three hours apart. Again, drink water BETWEEN meals and eat your protein FIRST.

For the seventh week following surgery and for the rest of your life, you will be eating solid food. Now you can slowly eat two ounces of protein and one to two ounces of carbohydrates (preferably vegetables) three to four times a day. Chew your food until it is mushy. These meals should be about five hours apart. Once again, drink liquids BETWEEN meals and eat your protein FIRST.

At this point and for the rest of the first year after your lap band surgery, you will be followed very closely. Why? Because, in order for the lap band to work, you need to feel restricted with your eating—not too little or too much, just the right amount. How do we know if you're restricted the right amount? Come into your doctor's office to find out.

If you don't get hungry, if you feel full after eating about one-half to one cup of food, if you can go about five hours between meals, if you have trouble swallowing bread and drier meats (trying to do this causes pressure in the middle of your chest), your band has the right amount of fluid in it.

If you're unable to eat solid food and instead drink fluids only (including high-calorie shakes), if you can barely tolerate swallowing liquids including your own saliva, if you vomit or regurgitate when you try to eat, your band is restricting you too much and some of the fluid needs to be removed.

If you feel hungry, if you can eat anything you want including bread and all kinds of meat, if you feel like you need to eat every couple of hours, your band is not restricting you and needs fluid added to it.

The amount of weight you are losing—or gaining—is also taken into consideration. But more emphasis is placed on how you're eating. There are foods that you may find you have a lot of trouble eating and should therefore avoid. These include

- ☹ Dry or stringy meat
- ☹ Calamari or shrimp
- ☹ Stringy or tough-skinned fruits and vegetables
- ☹ Doughy bread
- ☹ White rice or pasta—if you try this, eat it slowly

How to Eat Following the Roux-en-Y

While you are still in the hospital recovering from your surgery, you will be on a clear liquid diet. Clear liquids that you are allowed include coffee, tea, sugar-free gelatin, sugar-free fruit juices, and broth. Sip your liquids slowly and frequently. Your goal is to drink sixty-four ounces a day.

After you go home from the hospital, you will be eating soft foods for the next three months. Your meals should be up to four ounces serving size with good sources of protein. Make sure you eat slowly, taking very small bites and chewing your food well. You should eat three meals a day. And not to sound like a broken record, but drink your fluids BETWEEN meals, and eat your protein FIRST.

After the first three months and for the rest of your life, you will be eating solid food. Take very small bites and chew your food well. You should be able to eat one-half to one cup of food at each meal. Dare I say it again? Drink your fluids BETWEEN meals and eat your protein FIRST.

Biliopancreatic Diversion

How to Eat Following the BPD, *The Scopinaro Procedure*

While you are still in the hospital recovering from your surgery, you will be on a clear liquid diet. You will be asked to drink slowly but frequently. Remember, your goal is to get sixty-four ounces of fluid in every day.

After you go home from the hospital, you will be eating soft foods for the next two to four weeks. Be sure you are getting three small meals every day as well as two to three snacks throughout the day. Your meals should include two ounces of protein and one half cup (or less) of another food. And yes, for the hundredth time, drink your fluids BETWEEN meals and eat your protein FIRST.

After the first four weeks and for the rest of your life, you will be eating solid food. During the first few months after your surgery, you will probably find that you can only eat one-half to one cup of food at meals—similar to a patient who has undergone the Roux-en-Y. This is normal. After a few months, you should be able to eat larger meals. Remember to get your protein in first, especially since you need to get one hundred grams of protein in every day. Take smaller bites and chew your food well. And for the thousandth time, drink your fluids BETWEEN meals.

As you start getting used to your new (and permanent) eating habits, you may experience some problems like pressure in the middle of your chest, shoulder pain, or even the hiccups. You are probably eating too fast, eating too big a bite, or swallowing a lot of air. Try these suggestions:

☺   Be sure you are drinking fluids between meals, not with meals (has this been repeated enough?).

☺   Take small bites of food.

☺   Chew, chew, chew your food

☺   Take your time eating—similar to how you drank fluids before your surgery, you were probably used to taking big bites of food and eating fast—without even thinking about it; now you have to actually concentrate on chewing your food well; you may find that you have to avoid watching television or talking to someone while you eat so that you can concentrate.

☺   When you feel full, stop eating.

☺   If you don't experience the sensation of fullness but you feel chest pressure or you regurgitate your food, figure out how much food you can eat before those symptoms occur; the next time you eat, measure out that amount of food and stop eating when it is gone; this should prevent the chest pressure and regurgitation from occurring.

☺   When food feels stuck, try one capful of Coca Cola or one teaspoon of meat tenderizer; this will help the food break down enough to pass into your stomach.

One of the fears you may have after surgery is the possibility of regaining your weight. For the first year or so following your surgery, you may find you have no appetite. So eating small and infrequent meals is not such a big deal. And the number you see on the scale continues to go down or stabilizes. Then after that first year, your appetite returns. You may find yourself feeling like you need to eat more. It you are a lot more active (for example, exercising every day), you may need to be eating more. But you may start to regain weight, which is possible with all the bariatric surgeries.

It is actually normal to see your weight rebound. You may get down to your desired weight and then gain back ten maybe even twenty pounds. Part of this is your body telling you that it feels more comfortable at a higher weight—it's healthier at that higher weight. Try not to let this upset you. It is NORMAL for your body to do this. After you see the rebound in your weight, you should then see it stabilize. Aside from developing a good exercise program, here are some ways to prevent seeing the number creep up on your scale (once your weight has stabilized):

☺ Eat your protein-rich foods first (hmm . . . I think I've seen this before).

☺ Develop good eating habits from the get-go; this will be a very conscious effort at first; but eventually, your good eating habits will become just that—habits—things you do without thinking.

☺ Avoid watching television or carrying on conversations during the time that you are relearning how to eat; you will find that you really need to concentrate on taking small bites of food and chewing your food well; distractions make this more difficult to learn.

☺ Learn to recognize when you feel hungry and when you feel full; this will eventually become second nature to you.

☺ Don't sample food while you're cooking.

☺ Avoid high-calorie liquids (milkshakes, whole milk, full-fat cream soups, 2 percent milk, chocolate milk).

☺ Avoid high-fat breads and pastries (sweet rolls, doughnuts, pancakes, waffles, french toast, muffins, croissants).

☺ Avoid fried potatoes (french fries, potato chips, hash browns).

☺ Avoid high-fat proteins and meat (fried eggs, regular cheese, hotdogs, sausage, deep-fried meat, deep-fried poultry, deep-fried fish, bologna, pepperoni, salami, ribs, highly marbled meats).

☺ Be careful how you or others prepare vegetables (avoid fried, scalloped, or creamed vegetables).

☺ Avoid high-fat, crunchy foods (chips, cookies).

☺ Watch the kinds of desserts you choose (avoid cakes, cookies, brownies, ice cream, pies, puddings, custards, doughnuts, chocolate).

☺ Avoid grazing; eat only three meals a day and one or two snacks a day.

Another fear you may have following your surgery is that you will never be able to eat out at a restaurant again. But you can. You just need to be prepared when you go out. One of the first things you should do is mention to the waiter or waitress that you have undergone bariatric surgery. Show them your bariatric surgery card, if you have one. The next thing to do is ask if you can order off the menu ala carte, ordering just a breast of chicken or some other small portion of food. Many chain restaurants are more than happy to oblige, including the following:

☺ Applebee's

☺ Bravo's

- ☺   Brio
- ☺   Champs
- ☺   Cheesecake Factory
- ☺   Chili's
- ☺   Longhorn's Steakhouse
- ☺   Olive Garden
- ☺   Outback
- ☺   Texas Roadhouse

Family-owned and small-scale restaurants tend to be less willing to allow for you to order ala carte. When this happens, try to share a meal with someone else. You CAN enjoy dining out.

Okay! You're drinking plenty of water and fluids; you're eating right and getting your protein; now let's tackle vitamins.

VITAMINS AND OTHER NUTRIENTS

TAKING YOUR VITAMINS AND SUPPLEMENTS EVERY DAY?

Vitamins . . . vitamins . . . vitamins! Now it's time to make a big fuss about vitamins. Why do we worry so much about vitamins? Well, first of all, you're eating less. Before your surgery, you were able to eat larger quantities of food, so you were probably getting most of the vitamins and nutrients you needed from the foods you ate. Taking vitamins and supplements was probably not necessary. But now that you've had your surgery, your stomach pouch is smaller, and you are unable to eat as much. Therefore, you are not getting the vitamins and nutrients as before because you physically cannot eat the same quantity of food as before. Second, if you underwent one of the malabsorptive surgeries, that is, the Roux-en-Y or BPD, you're not absorbing your vitamins and nutrients from food as well so you must take your vitamin supplements every day.

Still not convinced that you need to take your vitamins? Just how important are they anyway? Let's look at various vitamins and nutrients and what they do for you and your body to keep you healthy. This is not an all-inclusive list, but many of the important ones are mentioned.

Iron. This is contained in blood. As blood travels through your lungs, oxygen attaches itself to iron. Why? This helps oxygen get carried to all parts of your body. And oxygen is necessary to provide energy and to keep the parts of your body alive.

Calcium. You've heard this before—calcium builds strong bones and teeth. But did you also know that it is essential for muscle contraction and the transmission of nerve impulses?

Vitamin D. This helps your body use calcium and phosphorus, which are necessary to build strong bones and teeth.

Vitamin B1 (Thiamin). This helps your body to use protein and carbohydrates to produce energy. It also helps with metabolism, especially of carbohydrates. It is also important for helping your nervous system function normally.

Vitamin B2 (Riboflavin). This can be found in every cell of your body. It is necessary for producing energy and is needed to help with metabolism and the function of skin and nerves.

Vitamin B3 (Niacin). This is found in every cell of your body. It is required for energy production as well as for making DNA. It also keeps your skin, nerves, and digestive system functioning as they should.

Vitamin B6 (Pyridoxine). This helps with regulating blood glucose (sugar) levels. It helps with the production of hemoglobin. It helps your body use protein, carbohydrates, and fats. And it helps with the function of your nervous system.

Vitamin B12. This is essential for normal growth, healthy nerve tissue, and the making of blood. It is crucial in the reproduction of every cell of the body.

Vitamin B9 (Folic Acid). This is needed for the manufacture of DNA, which is used in the reproduction of cells of your body. It helps with making red blood cells. It is also important for reducing the risks of certain birth defects in a developing fetus.

Pantothenic Acid. This is essential for the breakdown of fat and sugar in your body.

Zinc. This is needed for cell growth, cell reproduction, and cell repair. It helps with your body's immune response and the metabolism of insulin. It also helps with the healing of wounds.

There are other important vitamins and nutrients that you will need to supplement since you are eating less. They too have important roles in keeping your body healthy and functioning normally. They include the following:

Magnesium. This is necessary for the breakdown of glucose (sugar), the making of proteins and nucleic acids, muscle contraction, transmission of nerve impulses, and the delicate electrical balance of cells.

Phosphorus. This works with calcium to help with cell growth and with the making of your bones and teeth. It is also important in kidney function and the squeezing of your heart.

Potassium. This is essential for making all muscles function properly, including the heart. It is vital for the transmission of nerve impulses, digestion, and the release of insulin. It helps to maintain fluid balance between the inside and outside of cells.

Vitamin A. This is important for the growth and development of bones, teeth, and gums. It is essential for night vision, healthy skin, hair, and mucous membranes.

Vitamin C. This is an antioxidant. It helps with the formation of collagen (a protein found in the connective tissue of your skin, tendons, ligaments, bones, and cartilage), transmission of nerve impulses, and tissue repair.

Vitamin E. This is an antioxidant. It can prevent a process called oxidation, which can result in harmful effects in your body. It is important for the function of nerves and muscles.

Vitamin K. This helps blood clot when your body is injured. It is also important in bone metabolism.

Again, this is not an all-inclusive list of vitamins and nutrients, but they are some of the more common and more important ones you will hear about. As you are becoming accustomed to your new way of eating and the necessity of taking your vitamins, you may find yourself having trouble getting everything you need. If you're struggling, you may start to develop health problems. If you are having the following problems, you may not be getting enough of the vitamins or nutrients listed:

Anemia—Riboflavin, Vitamin B6, or Vitamin C

Bleeding gums—Riboflavin, Vitamin C, or Vitamin K

Blurry vision or **night blindness**—Vitamin A or Zinc

Bone tenderness—Calcium, Phosphorus, Vitamin C, or Vitamin D

Diarrhea—Folate, Niacin, or Vitamin B12

Edema (swelling)—Protein or Thiamin

Extremely dry eyes—Vitamin A

Hair loss, sparse or **thinning hair** or **hair that is easily pluckable***—Protein, Zinc, Biotin, or Linoleic acid

Impaired wound healing—Linoleic acid, Protein, Vitamin C, or Zinc

Irritability—Niacin, Thiamin, or Vitamin B6

Mental confusion—Niacin or Potassium

Muscle cramps, tenderness, or **pain**—Thiamin or Vitamin C

Muscle wasting—Protein

Muscle weakness—Potassium or Vitamin A

Nausea—Protein or Thiamin

Numbness, **tingling,** or **burning sensation**—Thiamin or Vitamin B6

Redness or **inflammation** of the **lips**, **tongue**, or **mouth**—Niacin, Riboflavin, or Vitamin B6

Skin rashes, **dermatitis**, **dry** and **scaling skin**—Essential fatty acids (Linoleic acid), Vitamin A, or Zinc

Weakness—Niacin, Riboflavin, Vitamin B6, or Vitamin C

*Hair loss that occurs early following your surgery is probably due to your rapid weight loss. As your weight stabilizes, you should stop losing hair and start to see it fill back in. Hair loss that occurs later on may be from a nutritional problem, especially iron deficiency. Other causes of hair loss include deficiencies in protein and zinc as mentioned above.

Daily Vitamin Recommendations for Lap Band

☺   One multivitamin or two chewable children's multivitamins

☺   Calcium citrate 1500 mg (500 mg three times a day)

☺   Zinc 50 mg

☺   Vitamin B12 (sublingual recommended) 500 mcg

Daily Vitamin Recommendations for Roux-en-Y

☺   One multivitamin with iron or two chewable children's multivitamins with iron

- ☺ Calcium citrate 1500 mg (500 mg three times a day)
- ☺ Zinc 50 mg
- ☺ Vitamin B12 (sublingual recommended) 500-1000 mcg
- ☺ Vitamin D 400 IU
- ☺ Iron 300 mg (150 mg two times a day, you will need a prescription)

You may choose to take a vitamin specifically formulated for bariatric patients who underwent the Roux-en-Y.

If you take Vita-4-Life, you will be recommended to take twelve tablets daily (four tablets three times a day) as well as an additional iron supplement.

Daily Vitamin Recommendations for BPD

- ☺ Two multivitamins with iron (one in am and one in pm) or four chewable children's multivitamins with iron (two in am and two in pm)
- ☺ Calcium citrate 1500 mg (500 mg three times a day)
- ☺ Zinc 50 mg
- ☺ Vitamin B12 (sublingual recommended) 1000 mcg
- ☺ Two Vitamin A and D tablets (one in am and one in pm) totaling Vitamin A 10,000 IU and Vitamin D 800 IU
- ☺ Iron 300 mg (150 mg two times a day, you will need a prescription)

Again, you may choose to take a vitamin specifically formulated for bariatric patients who underwent the BPD.

If you choose Vita-4-Life, you will be recommended to take twelve tablets daily (four tablets three times a day) as well as an additional iron supplement.

Following is a partial listing of some of the other brands of bariatric vitamins currently available. Some can be found in your local grocery store or pharmacy while others can be ordered over the Internet.

Bariatric Advantage
- ☺   Multivitamin, chewable
- ☺   Multivitamin, capsule
- ☺   VitaBand (for lap band patients)
- ☺   Calcium citrate
- ☺   Calcium crystals
- ☺   Vitamin B12, sublingual
- ☺   Iron, chewable
- ☺   Vitamin D, capsules

Bariatric Lifestyle
- ☺   Multivitamin, chewable

TwinLab
- ☺   Calcium citrate, chewable

Wonderlife
- ☺   Active Man's multivitamin
- ☺   Active Woman's multivitamin

☺   Multivitamin without iron, soft gel

☺   Super multivitamin, liquid

☺   Vitamin B12, sublingual

☺   Vitamin B6, tablets

☺   B complex

☺   Vitamin C

☺   Calcium and magnesium

☺   Calcium citrate and magnesium citrate

☺   Calcium citrate with vitamin D

☺   Osteo support formula

☺   Chelated Iron, tablets

☺   Zinc, tablets

☺   Fiber, capsules

When shopping for vitamins, read the labels carefully. Some vitamins are more potent than others, requiring you to take only one maybe two tablets. Vitamins with a lower potency may require you to take two or more tablets to get the recommended dose.

For the first few weeks after your surgery, you may find that the chewable forms of vitamins may be easier for you to take. Trying to swallow a vitamin the size of a horse pill may be too difficult. So how do you know which vitamin to choose? Well here are a couple of brands of chewable vitamins along with their specific vitamin and nutrient contents. You may prefer the taste of one over the other. Whichever vitamin you choose, make sure you are getting the required daily amounts based on the information given to you by your surgeon. Again, be aware of the sugar content. Not all vitamins are created equally.

The following is a comparison between the vitamin content of Centrum Chewables and Centrum Liquid.

Centrum	Chewable	Liquid (5.7% alcohol)
Serving size	1 tablet	1 tablespoon
Calories	5	25
Total carbohydrates	1 gram	5 grams
Sugar	Less than 1 gram	5 grams
Vitamin A	3500 IU	1300 IU
Vitamin C	60 mg	60 mg
Vitamin D	400 IU	400 IU
Vitamin E	30 IU	30 IU
Vitamin K	10 mcg	—
Thiamin	1.5 mg	1.5 mg
Riboflavin	1.7 mg	1.7 mg
Niacin	20 mg	20 mg
Vitamin B6	2 mg	2 mg
Folic acid	400 mcg	—
Vitamin B12	6 mcg	6 mcg
Biotin	45 mcg	300 mcg
Pantothenic acid	10 mg	10 mg
Calcium	108 mg	—

Iron	18 mg	9 mg
Phosphorus	50 mg	—
Iodine	150 mcg	150 mcg
Magnesium	40 mg	—
Zinc	15 mg	3 mg
Copper	2 mg	—
Manganese	1 mg	2 mg
Chromium	20 mcg	25 mcg
Molybdenum	20 mcg	25 mcg

The following is a comparison between the vitamin content of Flintstones Chewables and Flintstones Gummies.

Flintstones	Chewable	Gummies
Serving size	1 tablet	2 gummies
Calories	—	10
Total carbohydrates	Less than 1 gram	3 grams
Sugars	—	3 grams
Vitamin A	3000 IU	2000 IU
Vitamin C	60 mg	30 mg
Vitamin D	400 IU	200 IU
Vitamin E	30 IU	20 IU
Thiamin	1.5 mg	—
Riboflavin	1.7 mg	—
Niacin	15 mg	—
Vitamin B6	2 mg	1 mg

Folic acid	400 mcg	200 mcg
Vitamin B12	6 mcg	5 mcg
Biotin	40 mcg	75 mcg
Pantothenic acid	10 mg	5 mg
Calcium	100 mg	—
Iron	18 mg	—
Phosphorus	100 mg	—
Iodine	150 mcg	40 mcg
Magnesium	20 mg	—
Zinc	12 mg	2.5 mg
Copper	2 mg	—
Sodium	10 mg	—

There are also other formulations of the Flintstones vitamins, including Immunity Support, Bone Building Support, and Plus Iron. They are compared below:

	Immunity Support	Bone Building Support	Plus Iron
Serving size	1 tablet	1 tablet	1 tablet
Total carbs	< 1 gram	—	< 1 gram
Sugars	< 1 gram	—	< 1 gram
Vitamin A	2500 IU	2500 IU	2500 IU
Vitamin C	250 mg	60 mg	60 mg
Vitamin D	400 IU	400 IU	400 IU
Vitamin E	15 IU	15 IU	15 IU

Thiamin	1.05 mg	1.05 mg	1.05 mg
Riboflavin	1.2 mg	1.2 mg	1.2 mg
Niacin	13.5 mg	13.5 mg	13.5 mg
Vitamin B6	1.05 mg	1.05 mg	1.05 mg
Folic acid	300 mcg	300 mcg	300 mcg
Vitamin B12	4.5 mcg	4.5 mcg	4.5 mcg
Sodium	25 mg	10 mg	10 mg
Calcium	—	200 mg	—
Iron	—	—	15 mg

Vitamins won't be the only pills you take. In addition to the prescription medications you already take for blood pressure, diabetes, or other health problems, you will need to take an antacid. You will be asked to take this for at least six months after your surgery. You may say, "But I don't have reflux. Why do I have to take an antacid?" If you had the Roux-en-Y or BPD surgery, the part of your small intestine that is now attached to your stomach is not used to being exposed to stomach acid. With repeated exposure to the acid, an ulcer can form. Taking an antacid helps prevent ulcers from forming and allows the lining of your small intestine to toughen up. If after six months you don't have reflux, you will probably be able to stop taking your antacid as long as it is okay with your doctor.

Okay! You're taking your vitamin supplements and loving it! (Can I get a woohoo!) The information given next describes food sources, which also provide the necessary vitamins and nutrients you need.

The following tables contain dietary sources of iron: heme iron sources and nonheme iron sources. Heme iron sources are those that are absorbed much more easily by your body and are found in meat, fish, and poultry:

Food source	Serving size	Iron (mg)
Beef chuck	3 ounces	3.2
Beef flank	3 ounces	4.3
Beef liver	3 ounces	7.5
Beef round	3 ounces	4.6
Chicken breast	3 ounces	0.9
Chicken leg	2 ounces	0.7
Chicken liver	3 ounces	7.3
Chicken thigh	2.3 ounces	1.2
Cod, broiled	3 ounces	0.8
Corned beef	3 ounces	2.5
Flounder, baked	3 ounces	1.2
Ham, lean	3 ounces	1.9

Lean ground beef	3 ounces	3.9
Pink salmon, canned	3 ounces	0.7
Pork	3 ounces	1.9
Pork loin chop	3 ounces	3.5
Shrimp	1.1 ounce	0.5
Tuna, canned in water	3.5 ounces	1.0
Turkey, dark meat	3 ounces	2.0
Turkey, white meat	3 ounces	1.2

Nonheme iron sources are those found primarily in fruits, vegetables, dried beans, nuts, and grains:

Food source	Serving size	Iron (mg)
Almonds, raw	10-12	0.7
Apricots, dried	10	1.7
Bagel	1	1.5
Baked beans, canned	½ cup	2.0
Blackstrap molasses	1 tablespoon	2.3
Bread, white	2 slices	1.4
Bread, whole wheat	2 slices	1.7
Broccoli, cooked	½ cup	0.6
Broccoli, raw	1 stalk	1.1
Brown rice, cooked	1 cup	1.0
Dates	10	1.6
Kidney beans	½ cup	3.0
Lima beans	½ cup	1.8
Macaroni, enriched, cooked	1 cup	1.9

Peas, frozen	½ cup	1.3
Prune juice	½ cup	1.5
Raisins	¼ cup	1.0
Spaghetti, enriched, cooked	1 cup	1.6
Spinach, cooked	½ cup	2.0
White rice, enriched, cooked	1 cup	1.8

Calcium deficiency is often something that bariatric patients develop. There are many ways to increase the amount of calcium in your diet, for example,

☺   Milk and milk-based desserts like pudding, frozen yogurt, ice milk, and ice cream
☺   Cheese including soft cheeses, like ricotta and cottage cheese, and processed cheese like American cheese
☺   Yogurt
☺   Nondairy sources

Dairy sources of calcium and the milligrams of calcium in each serving include the following:

Source	Serving size	Calcium (mg)
1 percent milk	1 cup	300
2 percent milk	1 cup	295
Fat-free milk	1 cup	300
Oatmeal made with milk	1 cup	300

It is not unusual for you to develop lactose intolerance following your surgery, especially if you underwent the Roux-en-Y. If you do and you cannot drink milk or eat cheese or yogurt, getting the required calcium you need is not impossible. There are many nondairy foods that contain calcium. The following table lists these specific sources of calcium:

Source	Serving size	(mg)
Almonds	1 ounce	72
Blackstrap molasses	1 tablespoon	172
Broccoli, cooked	1 cup	71
Collards, cooked	1 cup	266
Cowpeas, cooked	½ cup	106
Dry cereal, calcium fortified	1 ounce	200-300
Kale, cooked	1 cup	90
Ocean perch	3 ounces	116
Orange juice, calcium fortified	1 cup	350
Other vegetables and most fruits	1 cup	10-60
Salmon with bones (no salt)	3 ounces	180
Sardines with bones (no salt)	3 ounces	325
Shrimp	3 ounces	45
Soymilk, calcium fortified	1 cup	350
Spinach	1 cup	291
Tofu with calcium	3 ounces	30-100
Turnip greens, cooked	½ cup	124

Vitamin D, another vitamin commonly found to be deficient in bariatric patients, is produced by your skin when you are exposed to sunlight. Depending on where you live, during the winter months, you may have a lot more gray days than sunny days. With less sunshine and therefore less vitamin D production by your body, it is very common to be deficient in vitamin D. Taking a vitamin supplement will help as will eating foods rich in vitamin D—going to Florida for a few weeks won't hurt either. Here are some dietary sources of Vitamin D (please note that the amount of vitamin D per serving is measured in international units or IU):

Food	Serving size	(IU)
Beef liver, cooked	3.5 ounces	15
Cereal, vitamin D fortified	¾-1 cup	40
Egg (with yolk)	1	20
Mackerel, cooked	3.5 ounces	345
Margarine, vitamin D fortified	1 tablespoon	60
Milk, vitamin D fortified	1 cup	98
Pudding, vitamin D fortified	½ cup	50
Pure cod liver oil	1 tablespoon	1360
Salmon, cooked	3.5 ounces	360
Sardines, canned in oil	1 ¾ ounces	250
Swiss cheese	1 ounce	12
Tuna fish, canned in oil	3 ounces	200

The B vitamins can be another source of deficiency in bariatric patients, especially vitamin B12. Dietary sources of all of the various B vitamins include the following:

Vitamin B1 (Thiamin)
Whole-grain cereals, bread, red meat, egg yolks, green leafy vegetables, legumes, sweet corn, brown rice, berries, yeast

Vitamin B2 (Riboflavin)
Whole-grain products, milk, meat, eggs, cheese, peas

Vitamin B3 (Niacin)
Protein-rich foods, meats, fish, brewer's yeast, milk, eggs, legumes, potatoes, peanuts

Vitamin B6 (Pyridoxine)
Liver, meat, brown rice, fish, butter, wheat germ, whole grain cereals, soybeans

Vitamin B12*
Liver, meat, egg yolk, poultry, milk
(See below for more specific food sources and the amount of vitamin B12 contained in each. Note the amount of vitamin B12 is measured in micrograms (μg).)

Vitamin B9 (Folic Acid)
Yeast, liver, green vegetables, whole-grain cereals

Pantothenic Acid

Meats, legumes, whole-grain cereals

*Food Sources of Vitamin B12

Food source	Serving size	(µg)
American cheese	1 ounce	0.3
Beef liver	1 slice	47.9
Breakfast cereals, 100 percent fortified	¾ cup	6.0
Breakfast cereals, 25 percent fortified	¾ cup	1.5
Chicken breast, roasted	½ breast	0.3
Clams, cooked	3 ounces	84.1
Egg, hard-boiled	1	0.6
Haddock, cooked	3 ounces	1.2
Ham	3 ounces	0.6
Milk	1 cup	0.9
Mollusks, cooked	3 ounces	84.1
Pork	3 ounces	0.6
Rainbow trout, farmed, cooked	3 ounces	4.2
Rainbow trout, wild, cooked	3 ounces	5.4
Salmon, cooked	3 ounces	4.9
Sockeye, cooked	3 ounces	4.9
Top sirloin beef, broiled	3 ounces	2.4
White tuna, canned in water	3 ounces	1.0
Yogurt, plain skim	1 cup	1.4

Zinc is often seen as a deficiency on routine lab work following bariatric surgery. Taking a supplement is recommended, but food can be a good way to get zinc too. Dietary sources of zinc include the following:

Food source	Serving size	Zinc (mg)
Alaskan king crab, cooked	3 ounces	6.5
Almonds, dry roasted	1 ounce	1.0
Baked beans, canned	½ cup	1.7
Beef shanks, cooked	3 ounces	8.9
Cashews, dry roasted	1 ounce	1.6
Cereal, fortified	¾ cup	3.8
Cheddar cheese	1 ounce	0.9
Chicken breast, roasted	½ breast	0.9
Chicken leg, roasted	1	2.7
Chickpeas	½ cup	1.3
Flounder, cooked	3 ounces	0.5
Kidney beans, cooked	½ cup	0.8
Lobster, cooked	3 ounces	2.5
Milk	1 cup	0.9
Mozzarella cheese	1 ounce	0.9
Oatmeal, instant	1 pack	0.8
Oysters	6 medium	76.7
Peas, boiled	½ cup	0.8
Pork shoulder, cooked	3 ounces	4.2
Pork tenderloin, cooked	3 ounces	2.5
Raisin bran	¾ cup	1.3
Sole, cooked	3 ounces	0.5

| Swiss cheese | 1 ounce | 1.1 |
| Yogurt, low fat with fruit | 1 cup | 1.6 |

In order to get the most from the vitamins you are taking, you need to make sure you are taking them properly. Here are some helpful tips to keep in mind:

- ☺ If you take a multivitamin and separate calcium supplement, remember that you should not take the calcium at the same time as the multivitamin, or the nutrients will not be absorbed properly.
- ☺ If you choose to take calcium, iron, and zinc as individual supplements, be sure to take each supplement at least thirty minutes apart from each other.
- ☺ Avoid taking your vitamins and supplements with caffeine as this can interfere with their absorption
- ☺ Take your vitamins at the same time every day—once this becomes a habit, you'll be less likely to forget taking them.
- ☺ Take your vitamins between meals—remember, your stomach pouch is small; if you take your vitamins (which you're probably taking with fluids) right before your meal, you won't be able to eat as much food as you need to.
- ☺ Powdered vitamins from GNC can be added to food (like yogurt); however, if you have had a BPD, you

            still need to take your vitamins in tablet form every day

☺   Celebrate brand chewable calcium may be more palatable to you; it is sold online and is a good price, but best of all, it comes in hot cocoa and strawberry cream flavors—yum!

Vitamins aren't the only things you may be deficient in after your surgery. It is not unusual to hear bariatric patients complain that they're not . . . you know . . . GOING as often. Now part of the reason for this is because you're not eating as much. Less food going in means less coming out. If you're not exercising, this can also contribute to constipation. Part of the reason for your constipation may be because you're not drinking enough. Dehydration can lead to constipation. If there isn't enough fluid to soften things up, the "trip out" becomes much more difficult. You may not be getting enough fiber or bulk in your diet, which works with your body to hold water in the intestinal tract, soften your stool, and increase the frequency of bowel movements.

There are two types of fiber: soluble and insoluble. Soluble fiber is a softer type of fiber and dissolves in water. It helps prevent cholesterol from being absorbed in your intestines and also helps to minimize rises in blood sugar levels after you eat. Soluble fiber can be found in foods like oat bran, oatmeal, some fruits, and some vegetables. Insoluble fiber doesn't dissolve in water. It's what works with your body to hold water in your intestinal tract, soften your stool, and increase the frequency of your bowel movements—it helps to keep your bowel movements regular. It is found in brown rice, bulgur, seeds, vegetables, wheat bran, and whole-wheat grain. If you think fiber may be lacking in your diet, here are some good food sources:

Food source	Serving size	Dietary fiber (gm)
Almonds	1 ounce	3.3
Apple with skin	1 medium	3.3
Artichoke, cooked	1 globe	6.5
Asian pear	1 small	4.4
Banana	1 medium	3.1
Black beans, cooked	½ cup	7.5
Blackberries	½ cup	3.8
Bran cereal 100 percent	½ cup	8.8
Broccoli, cooked	½ cup	2.8
Brussels sprouts, frozen	½ cup	3.2
Bulgur, cooked	½ cup	4.1
Chickpeas, cooked	½ cup	6.2
Collards, cooked	½ cup	2.7
Cowpeas, cooked	½ cup	5.6
Dates	¼ cup	3.6
Figs, dried	¼ cup	3.7

Great northern beans, cooked	½ cup	6.2
Green peas, cooked	½ cup	4.4
Guava	1 medium	3.0
Kidney beans, canned	½ cup	8.2
Lentils, cooked	½ cup	7.8
Lima beans, cooked	½ cup	6.6
Mixed vegetables, cooked	½ cup	4.0
Navy beans, cooked	½ cup	9.5
Oat bran muffin	1 small	3.0
Oat bran, raw	¼ cup	3.6
Okra, frozen	½ cup	2.6
Orange	1 medium	3.1
Parsnips, cooked	½ cup	2.8
Pinto beans, cooked	½ cup	7.7
Potato w/skin, baked	1 medium	3.8
Prunes, stewed	½ cup	3.8
Pumpkin, canned	½ cup	3.6
Raspberries	½ cup	4.0
Rye wafer crackers	2	5.0
Sauerkraut, canned	½ cup	3.0
Shredded wheat cereals	1 ounce	2.8-3.4
Soybeans, cooked	½ cup	5.2
Spinach, frozen	½ cup	3.5
Split peas, cooked	½ cup	8.1
Sweet potato w/ peel, cooked	1 medium	4.8
Sweet potato w/o peel, boiled	1 medium	3.9
Tomato paste	¼ cup	2.9

Turnip greens, cooked	½ cup	2.5
White beans, canned	½ cup	6.3
Whole-wheat English muffin	1	4.4
Whole-wheat spaghetti, cooked	½ cup	3.1
Winter squash, cooked	½ cup	2.9

Let's see; you're drinking plenty of water and fluids; you're eating right and getting your protein; you're taking all of your vitamins. What's next? Exercise.

EXERCISE

TAKING TIME TO EXERCISE THIRTY MINUTES EVERY DAY?

Exercise . . . exercise . . . exercise! You've heard about it. You know you should be doing it. It's time to start sweating! Yeah, sure you'll lose weight just with your new eating habits. But if you want to see even better weight loss, then you've got to exercise. Exercise will help you achieve your weight loss goals even faster. But not only that, exercise will help you maintain your bone density, increase your strength and balance, boost your energy level, improve your mood, and overall make the quality of your life better. People who exercise regularly tend to get sick less. Exercise also releases chemicals called endorphins, which give you a natural feeling of well-being.

You may be thinking, *That's all fine and good. But what do you suggest I do? Do you expect me to just go to a gym and work out?* The answer would be choose what suits you best. Exercise at home, exercise in a gym, or exercise with a personal trainer in a personal training studio. The bottom line is it's important for you to increase your physical activity.

You've been dealing with your obesity for some time now, and you're more painfully aware than anyone else of how difficult it may be for you to exercise. Let's face it; many of the machines and pieces of equipment at gyms aren't designed to accommodate obese people. Weight benches are too narrow. Seats on the machines are often too small. Until you've lost some weight, lying on your back to do exercises may be impossible if you have breathing problems.

Trying to do abdominal crunches may be difficult because of the size of your belly. Doing lunges and squats may cause too much pain in your knees. You've probably heard how great water aerobics is for toning muscles and losing weight. But unless you've lost a lot of weight—which may be true if you're further out from your surgery—showing yourself in public with just your bathing suit on may be more than you want to deal with.

There are some solutions to these problems. One of the first things you need to do, though, is decide you WILL exercise. Following are some tips to not only help you get started exercising but to keep you motivated to continue exercising for the rest of your life:

- ☺ Choose activities that are fun to you—if the activities are fun, you're more likely to keep doing them.
- ☺ Vary the type of exercise or activity you do—this will help keep you interested and make your exercises less boring.
- ☺ Make an appointment with yourself to exercise—pick a place and time to do your daily exercise or activity; be sure to keep your daily appointment; this is something you need to do for yourself.
- ☺ Start out exercising three days of the week; as you can do more, increase the number of days per week you exercise and the amount of time you spend exercising;

current guidelines recommend exercising at least thirty minutes a day for most days of the week.

☺ Listen to your favorite music while you exercise—music can be very motivating and energizing.

☺ Surround yourself with people who are supportive of your exercising—include your spouse, kids, friends, and coworkers in your activities; having a workout buddy will keep you focused and motivated

☺ Set goals for yourself—start small, walking for five minutes a day, and progress to greater duration and intensity, walking thirty minutes a day; write down your goals and share them with your family and friends; you're more likely to be held accountable if you do.

☺ Start slowly—don't try to keep up with the marathon runner; do what you are physically able to do and progress to more difficulty as you can; this will help you avoid injury.

☺ Keep a record of your activities—this not only can be motivating, but it also allows you to see what activities you've done and what new things you can try.

☺ Be flexible with the routine you set up for yourself—you may be too tired or feel too sick to do your exercise on a certain day; that's okay; give yourself the break you need but be sure to get right back on track before you lose your motivation.

The following are some simple ways to incorporate exercise into your daily life. Some of these can be done without even breaking a sweat:

☺ Get up thirty minutes earlier in the morning to do your exercising—yeah, you heard me; get up early! Have you told yourself you will exercise when you get home from work, and then you get home from work and say to yourself, "What? Are you nuts? You want me to exercise now? I'm too tired!" Get up first thing in the morning when you have plenty of energy—and fewer excuses—and get it done! Exercising in the morning not only gives you more energy to get you through your day, but it also boosts your metabolism.

☺ Take your (or someone else's) dog for a walk.

☺ Clean your house—this can burn a lot of calories, from scrubbing the floors to running the vacuum cleaner.

☺ Walk or ride your bike to pick up that small purchase at the store down the street.

☺ Go for a short walk before breakfast, after dinner, or both.

☺ Work in the garden or rake leaves or mow the grass—and not with a riding mower!

☺ Go to the mall and window-shop.

☺ Park farther out in the parking lot and walk the extra distance.

☺   Take the stairs instead of the elevator or escalator.

☺   Ride a stationary bike or use hand weights while you watch television.

☺   Get up to change the television station instead of using the remote control.

☺   Stand up and walk around while you talk on the telephone.

☺   Sometime during your workday, take a ten-minute walk—either at lunch or break time.

☺   Take a walk with a coworker while you dream up new project ideas.

☺   Walk down the hall to talk to someone rather than pick up the telephone.

☺   Take up dancing—you could be the next superstar of Dancing with the Stars.

☺   Join a softball team, soccer team, or bowling league or start one of your own.

☺   Join a fitness club—you may stick with this because of the cost involved.

☺   Join your local YMCA.

You are ready to start your exercise program now, but what kind of exercise do you want to do? There are two types of exercise you can do: aerobic and anaerobic. With aerobic exercise, your body uses oxygen to break down glucose (sugar). This provides the fuel needed by your body to produce energy to perform such activities as walking, jogging, running, and swimming. Aerobic exercises burn about 25 percent muscle and 75 percent fat and give you an overall cardiovascular workout.

With anaerobic exercises, your body doesn't require oxygen to create energy and includes resistance training and weight lifting. Anaerobic exercises burn 100 percent fat. Anaerobic exercise burns more calories than aerobic exercise at a ratio of 5 to 1, according to some sources. So bring on the weights! When doing weight lifting and resistance training, be sure to rotate muscle groups each time, working upper body one day and lower body the next time. This will allow your muscles to repair themselves, which strengthens and builds them.

If you are someone who has knee, hip, back, or other joint problems and walking across a room causes severe pain, exercising may seem completely out of the question. But it's not. There is a fitness program known as IsoBreathing that is specifically designed for morbidly obese people who have physical limitations. It involves a combination of isometrics—a muscle contraction that is maintained—and slow, rhythmic breathing. Most of the exercises can be done while seated on a chair. Part of the program incorporates the use of the IsoBand resistance band. You can improve your flexibility, endurance, range of motion, and strength—and lose weight—doing this exercise program. Check out the IsoBreathing.com Web site for more information or to buy this in-home workout program.

You may find that until you've lost a lot of weight, you feel too self-conscious to exercise at a gym or YMCA. You would feel much more comfortable exercising in the privacy of your own home. Are you unsure of how to make this happen? Here are some lower-cost suggestions to help you get started at home. Remember to start slow, and if at any time you feel pain in your joints when you are exercising, stop immediately. If you feel burning in your muscles while exercising, keep going—your muscles are telling you that you're doing it right.

Hand weights—these can be store-bought or homemade. For less expensive hand weights, try using water bottles, canned goods, or small liquid laundry detergent or fabric softener bottles. If you use the bottles, start with them empty until you are comfortable with the exercise you are doing, and then add a cup of water to each bottle to add more weight and resistance. As you can tolerate more weight, add another cup of water to each bottle. Keep doing this until the bottles are full.

If you have the money and are willing to spend it on exercise equipment for your home, recumbent bikes or recumbent cross-trainers are options. These allow you to get an effective workout without stressing your joints. Other options for home exercise equipment include a portable peddler or an exercise ball. Sitting on an exercise ball helps you improve your balance, improve your stability, and strengthen your abdominal muscles. You can also try marching while sitting on the ball, lifting one foot up at a time.

Once you're feeling stronger and you're not as physically limited by pain, fatigue, and shortness of breath, you're ready to progress to exercises that require you to be on your feet. It is very important to follow proper technique in order to prevent injury while exercising. So look to an experienced instructor for help. If you exercise at home, however, guidance from an exercise physiologist or instructor is not readily available. One solution is to buy workout programs on DVD (or VHS)—you may have seen infomercials for various programs on television. However, cost may again be an issue as some of the programs can be expensive to buy.

Beachbody is a popular source for exercise programs and can be found by going to their Web site Beachbody.com. Each of their exercise programs provides great guidance regarding proper technique. In many of the workouts, there is someone demonstrating beginner moves or modified moves that you can follow along with until you are stronger and able to do more. The instructors are very motivational, and their workouts are fun yet challenging. If you choose to buy a workout program through this Web site, the necessary equipment for these workouts often comes with the program when you order it (like weighted hand gloves, stability or exercise balls, and resistance bands). Items like hand weights and yoga mats will need to be purchased separately.

The following programs are currently available through the Beachbody Web site:

(Beachbody and the names of the Beachbody products are used with permission.)

Tony Horton

Program	Description
10 Minute Trainer	Ten-minute workouts that combine fat-burning cardio moves, total body toning and sculpting, and abdominal workouts; uses resistance bands
Power 90	Cardio-and-body-sculpting workouts using cardio, kickboxing, and Pilates; uses resistance bands
P90X	Twelve extreme workouts including muscle strengthening, cardio, yoga, and abdominals that can be mixed and matched in many ways to create a one-hour workout
P90X Plus	Incorporates advanced cardio and muscle strengthening
Power 90 Master Series	Incorporates advanced cardio-and-sculpting workouts
Power Half Hour	Combines cardio and targeted body sculpting
One-on-one with Tony Horton	Volume 1, Disc 4 Just Arms

| Tony and the Kids! | Combines stretching, hopping, jumping, kicking, and twisting |
| Tony and the Folks! | Thirty-minute low-impact workouts for people age fifty-five and up |

Chalene Johnson

Program	Description
Turbo Jam Maximum Results	Kickboxing and body sculpting set to fun and motivational music; incorporates dance and martial arts moves; some workouts use weighted hand gloves or light weights
Turbo Jam Fat Burning Elite	Incorporates advanced kickboxing and body sculpting
Turbo Jam Live!	Combines kickboxing and body sculpting; some workouts use light weights
Chalene Johnson's Get on the Ball!	Cardio and abdominal workout using a stability ball
ChaLEAN Extreme	Circuit training combining cardio and resistance training; uses heavy weights

Speaking from experience, these workouts are FUN, FUN, FUN! I truly look forward to doing her workouts. The music is very upbeat, and as you get more familiar with the workouts, you tend to get lost in the music. Chalene Johnson is a very inspirational and enthusiastic instructor.

Debbie Siebers

Program	Description
Slim in 6	Combines cardio with light resistance to burn fat and sculpt your entire body; uses light weights and resistance bands
Slim Series	More intense cardio and greater resistance
Slim Series Express	More intense cardio and greater resistance
Total Body Solution	With Chad Waterbury; fifteen-minute workouts designed to alleviate pain, stiffness, and injuries of the neck, shoulders, abdominals/core, lower back, and knees
Great Body Guaranteed!	With Tony Horton; five workouts each under ten minutes; designed to target a different area of your body

Shaun T

Program	Description
Hip Hop Abs	Dance moves designed to trim and give definition to abdominals without doing crunches; overall body workout

Hip Hop Abs Ultimate Results	Cardio and full-body sculpting
Rockin' Body	Cardio and full-body sculpting
Shaun T's Dance Party Series	Cardio and full-body sculpting
Get Real With Shaun T™	Alternates cardio and strength training
Shaun T's Fit Kids DVD	Light cardio for kids

Yoga Booty Ballet

Program	Description
Yoga Booty Ballet	Combines yoga, dance, and body sculpting; uses light weights
Yoga Booty Ballet Master Series	Combines yoga and Pilates
Yoga Booty Ballet Live!	Combines dance and body sculpting

Kathy Smith

Program	Description
Project: You! Type 2!™	Workouts designed especially for people trying to prevent or control Type 2 diabetes; this is another program that is ideal for people just starting out exercising

Again, cost may be an issue for you. If it is, try one of the following ideas:

- ☺ Go to your library and borrow the DVD (or VHS) of the program you are interested in trying; it's free, and it gives you a chance to see if the workout is right for you before you purchase it.
- ☺ Go to a used bookstore (Half-Price Books, for example) or check out EBay; you can find many different workout programs—including those seen in infomercials—for very little money; be careful when shopping Internet sites as illegal, counterfeit, and pirated copies of videos and disks may be out there lurking.

The following are seven of the most effective exercises you can do to help take and keep your weight off. You can do these on your own at home or in a gym with the guidance of a trainer. These exercises can also be found incorporated into programs available on DVD (or VHS):

- ☺ Walking—start out walking for only five minutes a day; as you can tolerate it, add more minutes to your walk until you are doing a minimum of thirty minutes at a time
- ☺ Interval training—this involves aerobic activity (swimming, biking, walking, running, etc.); with this type of training, you have short one-to-two-minute

bursts of higher intensity (for example, bicycling harder or with more resistance) followed by longer two-to-ten-minute segments of lesser intensity

☺   Squats—multiple major muscle groups of the lower body are worked simultaneously, which will help you burn more fat and calories; try using a chair to help you keep your balance (as needed)

☺   Lunges—multiple major muscle groups of the lower body are worked simultaneously with these too, helping you burn more fat and calories

☺   Push-ups—muscles of the chest, shoulders, triceps, and core (abdominal muscles and back muscles) are worked simultaneously; start out doing these on your knees; if you can only do one at first, don't worry; as you get stronger, you will be able to do more

☺   Abdominal crunches—there are many ways to do these (lying down or standing)

☺   Bent over row—muscles of the upper back and biceps are worked at the same time

You may prefer to join a gym rather than exercise at home. If you do get a gym membership, you may find that you're more likely to go if you have someone to go with you, like your spouse, your bother or sister, your friends, your coworkers, or other bariatric patients. You may even choose to take your kids with you. If you decide to join a gym, be sure to do your homework.

How structured a workout do you want? Many facilities will offer a personal trainer to guide you in choosing the best exercises, as well as help you do each exercise correctly using proper body mechanics. Some facilities, like Curves, give more guidance and structure to your routine. Find out if you will be charged extra for a personal trainer or if it is part of your membership fee.

And speaking of membership fees, compare the cost of different facilities. What are the basic features of the gym's membership? Are there any amenities? Make sure you are comfortable with the gym you want to join. If they're pushy about getting you to join when you're just trying to get information, how are they going to treat you after you're a member?

Do you feel comfortable exercising at a coed facility? Would you feel more comfortable going to a gym just for women? Other things to consider are time and travel. How far are you willing to drive to get to the gym? Do you want to pick a place close to home or close to work? Would you prefer your gym to be within walking distance or driving distance? Be sure you know the hours of operation. If you want to be that early bird who gets your workout done first thing in the morning, will the gym you choose be open at an early hour?

No matter what type of exercises you choose to do, make sure you keep water nearby. You will need to stay hydrated throughout your workout (remember, muscles like water). Plain water is best, but flavored water or LOW-calorie water is okay too.

Wow! You're drinking plenty of water and fluids; you're eating right and getting your protein; you're taking all of your vitamins; you're exercising every day; what kind of complications or problems are you having? Let's take a look.

COMPLICATIONS

Any Problems Since Your Surgery?

You've gone through your surgery, and things are running along smoothly. You're starting to get used to your new lifestyle; then you hit a bump in the road. What happened? Did something go wrong with your surgery? Did you do something wrong? Is there something that could have been done to prevent this problem from happening? What do you do now?

There are complications and problems that can occur immediately following or very soon after your surgery, even while you are still in the hospital. These are not all of the complications or problems that can happen, but many are talked about.

Anastomotic Leak

If you had the Roux-en-Y or BPD (switch) surgery, during your procedure different areas of your small intestine and stomach were divided and sewn back together. This was done in a few areas. The place where the stomach or small intestine was cut and then stapled and/or stitched back together again is called an anastomosis. The first anastomosis was made where the stomach and small intestine were brought together, and the second anastomosis was made where the small intestine and small intestine were brought together. It is at these spots where leaks can occur. What exactly leaks out, and why is it important? The fluids you drink and foods you eat may be in your stomach or small intestine. With the food and fluid is stomach acid. If the place where things are put back together has a leak, then the contents of your stomach or small intestine, which is partially digested food, leak out and go into your belly. This can cause inflammation, infection, belly pain, and a feeling of being bloated. Common symptoms of a leak are fevers and chills, sweating, fast heart rate, breathing fast, dehydration, and kidney problems that cause you to pee less. Fortunately, leaks don't happen very often. In fact, they rarely occur after the first two weeks of surgery.

Bowel Obstruction

A bowel obstruction is a blockage in your intestine that prevents digested food from traveling through. This can occur shortly after surgery and can be caused by an internal hernia (which we discuss later on), kinking at the place where the small intestine was sewn to the small intestine or complete closure where they're sewn together, twisting of the intestines or scar tissue. Symptoms that you may have early on include nausea and vomiting, and you may even have problems drinking fluids. You may or may not have belly pain. If your doctor suspects you have an obstruction, he or she will want to fix it right away in the operating room. A bowel obstruction is not a common problem, so don't get too nervous thinking about it.

Fatigue

If you're feeling really tired after your surgery, well, you should. You just went through major surgery. The tiredness you feel should only last for about one to two weeks if you had the lap band surgery and about four to eight weeks if you had the Roux-en-Y or BPD surgery. You may get your energy back sooner than others; you may even get your energy back later than others. Just keep in mind that it shouldn't last a long time. Be sure to rest when you need to.

Nausea and Vomiting

Nausea and vomiting are very common problems that can be seen after any surgery. Anesthesia medications and pain medications can cause you to feel nauseous. While you are in the hospital, you are given medication, either through your IV or by mouth, which helps to prevent or take away nausea and vomiting. When you go home from the hospital, you are given a prescription for medication that helps you avoid or, if you already have it, take away your nausea and vomiting. As you will read, there are many other problems that can cause nausea and vomiting too.

Pulmonary Embolus

A blood clot to your lungs, or pulmonary embolus (abbreviated PE), can occur after your surgery. The blood clot usually starts in a deep vein in one of your legs and then travels to your lungs. If you have a blood clot in your leg, your leg usually becomes swollen; and when you or someone else tries to push your toes up toward your nose, it hurts. Symptoms of a PE include feeling short of breath, breathing faster than normal, pain in your chest, cough, pain in your leg(s)—which is caused by the blood clot—coughing up blood, feeling your heartbeat racing, and wheezing. Signs that your doctor will look for to decide if you have a pulmonary embolus include a really fast heart rate, a really fast breathing rate, a crackling sound in your lungs, extra heart sounds, signs of a blood clot in your leg, and elevated temperature. Rest assured that your surgeon does everything that can be done to prevent the blood clots from forming in the first place. Your doctor will put you on blood thinners, get you up out of bed, and have you move around soon after your surgery and will have you wear those funny sequential compression devices (or SCDs) that periodically squeeze your lower legs. And you thought you wore those just to get a massage!

Pneumonia

While you are still in the hospital and for a short time after you go home, you will be asked to use a handheld breathing device, also known as a spirometer, to practice deep breathing. Why do your doctor and your nurse in the hospital care if you use your spirometer? If you don't breathe deeply, your lungs may not inflate completely. By breathing deeply, you pop open all those tiny air sacs in your lungs, which will help you to breathe better overall. The other reason is when you breathe deeply using the spirometer, it causes you to cough. While coughing is about the last thing you want to do since it only aggravates any pain or discomfort you may be having along your incision, it does a wonderful thing for you. It causes you to force out of your lungs any yucky stuff that may be sitting in there thinking, *This place is great! Warm, moist, nothing going on! I can grow like gangbusters down here!* Get that yucky stuff out of there. You really don't want to get pneumonia; I mean face it; it will only make you feel bad, and your recovery from surgery will be that much harder.

Death

Yikes! Do we really have to talk about this? Well, just be aware that it is something that happens, albeit rarely. The best thing you can do to prevent this from happening is to tell your doctor of any problems you are having, especially anything that doesn't seem normal or right to you. These could be warning signs of more serious problems. For example, some nausea and vomiting after surgery is not unusual. But if it seems like you're vomiting all the time, that's a problem. If you're having pain along your incision or mild abdominal pain after your surgery, this is probably nothing to worry about. But if you're having abdominal pain long after your surgery, especially severe pain, that's a different story. If you're not sure the problem you're having is important enough to mention to your doctor, just ask.

There are other problems that can occur after you've gone home from the hospital. Some of these problems can occur within the first week after surgery. Other problems can occur years after your surgery.

Bad Breath

This is an easy one to fix. First of all, are you brushing your teeth? Good. Are you drinking sixty-four ounces of water every day? Excellent. Maybe the problem is your stomach pouch. One thing you can do to help prevent bad breath is make sure you are taking your antacid. This should help. Another problem could be that you're not getting enough protein. During the first year or so after your surgery, your body is losing weight rapidly and is breaking down protein (muscles). This process is known as ketosis. When this happens, your breath may smell sweet (kind of a sickening sweet smell). You can help prevent the breakdown of your muscles by making sure you are eating and drinking enough protein.

Constipation

First of all, are you sure you're constipated? If you are having bowel movements every other day or every three days instead of every day and they are soft, you are not constipated. If you are having one or fewer bowel movements per week, then you are constipated. If your stool is hard, then you are constipated. If you are still taking pain medications, especially narcotic pain medications, these can cause constipation. Are you drinking sixty-four ounces of water every day (can you believe I'm still bugging you about this)? Increasing your fluids will help prevent constipation. Are you getting enough fiber in your diet? In addition to the foods mentioned in chapter 3 that contain higher amounts of fiber, you can try powders like Benefiber, Citrucel, and Metamucil. You can also try milk of magnesia, stool softeners, suppositories, or enemas. All of these items are available to you over the counter at your pharmacy.

Dehydration

Did you read chapter 1 "Fluids and Drinking Habits"? Good. Then you shouldn't become dehydrated. However, if you don't drink enough water and other fluids, these are some of the symptoms you may experience: mild dehydration is sometimes associated with a fast heart rate; moderate dehydration can be associated with dry skin, dry mucous membranes, and fast heart rate.

Fatigue

If you're feeling tired long after you should have recovered from your surgery, you may have anemia or vitamin B12 deficiency. Let your health care provider know that you're feeling tired so that labs can be ordered. You may need to increase your iron levels either through iron infusions or doubling up on your iron pills. You may need to undergo B12 injections or increase the amount of the vitamin B12 you're taking. If your anemia is severe enough, you may need a blood transfusion (this can occur with a bleeding ulcer).

Nausea and Vomiting

You hoped this was only a problem right after surgery, but unfortunately, it can happen later on down the road. While you're still taking pain medication, you can have nausea and vomiting. The nausea and vomiting could also be a result of dumping syndrome, a bowel obstruction, an ulcer, or even low blood sugar. If you're not eating or drinking enough protein, you can get nauseated from this.

Unfortunately, when you do feel nauseated from too little protein intake, you don't feel like eating. When you don't feel like eating, you don't get your protein in. When you don't get your protein in, you feel more nauseated. Do you see the vicious cycle this creates? Ugh!

There a few things you can do to prevent this cycle from starting: take your antacid (Nexium, Protonix, or whatever you were prescribed) every day; when you start to feel nauseous, take your nausea medication; when the nausea settles down, EAT! But be careful how you eat, because—guess what?—if you eat too fast, this can make you vomit too! You didn't think eating would be this much of a challenge? Well, it's really not. Just listen to your body; it knows how to tell you when you're hungry, when you're satisfied and don't need to eat anymore, and when you've eaten one bite too many. Pay attention to your body's cues; you'll be fine.

Too Much Weight Loss

Are you kidding? You can lose TOO much weight with bariatric surgery? Why yes, you can. Granted it doesn't happen very often, but it can happen. If you're vomiting all the time, you can lose too much weight. If you don't have much of or any appetite and you forget to eat, you can lose too much weight. If you had the lap band procedure and your band is so tight that you cannot eat and you can barely swallow your own saliva, you can lose too much weight. If you had the BPD surgery and your body is not absorbing enough protein, you can lose too much weight. Be sure to let your surgeon know if any of these problems are happening.

Weight Regain

You may have heard this from other people: you can regain weight after your surgery, and it doesn't matter if you had the lap band, Roux-en-Y, or BPD. You can even regain so much weight that you end up back where you started before your surgery. If you eat or drink the wrong things, graze or don't exercise, you can gain back a lot of weight. The most common causes of weight gain include eating sweets and drinking regular pop. To learn more about weight regain and how to prevent it from happening, see chapter 2 "Protein and Eating Habits."

Wound Infection

One of the bad things about being obese and undergoing surgery, any surgery, is that you are at higher risk of developing an infection of your incisions. If you are diabetic, this can add to your risk of getting an infection too. What can you do? Keep your incisions clean and dry. When you take a shower, get your hands soapy and rub them along your incisions; then just rinse under the shower of water. Try to avoid using a washcloth on your incisions because it can be too abrasive.

You know those annoying scabs on your incisions that you just want to pick off? Leave them there! Those scabs are protecting your incisions. When they're ready, they'll fall off. And when all your scabs have fallen off, then you can apply vitamin E or some other scar minimizing cream to your incisions. If you apply lotions and creams to your incisions before the scabs have fallen off, the creams can get under the scabs and into your incisions and cause—you guessed it—an infection.

So be patient and give your cuts time to heal. If you think you have an infection, let your health care provider know right away. Signs and symptoms of infection include redness along your incisions, drainage that appears cloudy or smells bad, increased pain along your incisions, and fever.

Complications Unique to Lap Band Patients

Esophageal Dilatation

The esophagus is made of muscles, and the muscles help to send food down into your stomach when you eat. After lap band surgery, the pouch where food is sent is much smaller. This creates resistance above the stomach pouch. Sometimes it takes more pushing by the esophagus to get the food to go into the stomach pouch. When this happens, the muscles of the esophagus can lose their tone and get stretched. To fix this, fluid is removed from your band to make the opening from the stomach pouch to the rest of your stomach bigger. This decreases the amount of resistance on the esophagus to send food down. With time, the part of the esophagus that was stretched can usually fix itself. Once this is resolved, you can have fluid put back into your band.

Long-term Erosion

When there is too much rubbing or friction of the band against your stomach over a long period of time, the band can actually cause a hole or erosion in your stomach. One way to tell if you have an erosion is if the incision over your port becomes infected long after your surgery. When you develop an erosion, the only thing to do is to take out your band and repair your stomach. A new band does not get placed at the same time the erosion is repaired. The erosion causes infection, and it's never a good idea to put a fresh, clean band in an area that's infected. Why? Because the new band can become infected too. A new band can be placed several months after the stomach has been fixed and is healed. Fortunately, this problem does not happen very often at all anymore. The newer bands that are being used by your surgeon are designed better than the older bands. The newer design helps prevent an erosion from occurring.

Slippage

The band may slide up or down, which can lead to problems. This complication doesn't take place very much either. After your band is positioned around your stomach, it is secured in place by taking stomach below your band and sewing it to stomach above the band. This is done in a few spots and makes it much more difficult for your band to move up, down, and around.

Complications Unique to Roux-En-Y Patients

Cholecystitis or Cholelithiasis

Those are fancy words that just mean your gallbladder is either inflamed or has stones in it. How does this happen, and what does the gallbladder do? The gallbladder stores and releases bile—a fluid made by the liver. Bile helps to break down fats in the foods you eat. Normally, after you eat, the gallbladder squeezes bile into ducts (small tubes); and the bile then travels to your small intestine where it helps with digestion. When stones form in your gallbladder, they can prevent bile from flowing out like it should, causing pain and other problems. If you've had the BPD (switch), then your gallbladder was removed during your surgery, you don't have to worry about this. After Roux-en-Y surgery, you're losing weight rapidly. This can cause gallstones to form. The stones can block the ducts (or tubes) that drain bile from your gallbladder. This causes pain and inflammation. The pain is usually felt in the right upper side of your belly. You may also experience pain in your shoulder blade, back or below your breastbone. What happens next? Your gallbladder needs to come out in surgery.

Dumping Syndrome

If you've suffered from nausea, bloating, belly pain, diarrhea, lightheadedness, diaphoresis (breaking out in a sweat), or palpitations after eating a meal high in sugar or fat, you've probably experienced dumping syndrome. Why does this happen? The part of your small intestine that is now directly attached to your stomach is not used to getting undigested food. It's used to the food that's well digested. Food particles cause extra fluid to rush to this area of the small intestine, and this makes you feel lousy. The sugar causes a lot of insulin to be released, which makes your blood sugar drop tremendously low. Low blood sugar will cause the symptoms mentioned. Many bariatric patients find that they can still eat sweets after surgery, but they learn from experience just how much they can eat before their symptoms start.

Gastrogastric Fistula

Gastro—what? This is a connection that develops between your tiny stomach pouch and the rest of your old stomach. During your surgery, your stomach is cut into two pieces: a tiny pouch and a large remnant stomach. Your stomach pouch is small and is where your food goes when you eat. The rest of your stomach is big and remains attached to the part of your small intestine that was bypassed. But the small stomach pouch and the big stomach remnant are not attached. The big remnant, as it is called, does not have food coming to it anymore. It still has its blood supply and nerve supply to continue secretion of digestive juices. How does the connection between the pouch and remnant develop? If you develop an ulcer, particularly a marginal ulcer, and the ulcer causes a lot of inflammation, this area can attach to the big stomach remnant and create a connection. It's also possible that your stomach pouch can migrate close to the big stomach remnant and reattach itself—for no reason at all. If a fistula, or connection, develops, you may stop losing weight or gain weight after you've been losing weight. Nausea, vomiting, and frequent upper belly pain can also occur.

Problems Unique to BPD (Switch) Patients

Multiple Bowel Movements and Foul-Smelling Stool and Gas

It won't be unusual for you to have four to eight loose bowel movements a day early after your surgery. You will also have more gas and more foul-smelling stool. Why? You have more gas because you are chewing more and swallowing more air when you chew. You are also swallowing smaller and more bites of food, which also causes you to swallow more air. Why does your stool smell foul? Before your surgery, your food was getting broken down and digested in the stomach and first part of your small intestine. But since these areas were bypassed in your surgery, food that is undigested or partially digested is coming through. When it reaches the colon, it is decomposed by the bacteria resulting in foul-smelling stool. Whew! There are deodorizers you can buy and carry with you that can mask the odor. Also remember, with regard to the number of trips to the bathroom, what you eat and the length of your common channel (the portion of the small intestine not bypassed in your surgery) will affect how often you visit the bathroom and how foul smelling your stool will be. If you eat a meal that is high in fat, be prepared to make extra trips to the bathroom and carry extra deodorizer.

Complications Seen in Both Roux-en-Y and BPD (Switch) Patients

Bowel Obstruction

This can occur later on after your surgery, long after you've gone home from the hospital. It can be associated with an internal hernia (which is explained later) or scar tissue. If you have pain around your belly button that comes and goes, it may be because of a bowel obstruction. You may also have symptoms of vomiting and bloating. Talk to your surgeon if you are having these symptoms.

Hernias

There are two different kinds of hernias we'll talk about: internal hernias and incisional hernias. Both types of hernias usually occur later after your surgery.

Internal hernias are those that can occur deep inside your belly. During your surgery, holes are made in fat that connect different parts of your small and large intestines. This allows for rerouting of your small intestines. However, if these holes are not fixed (usually by sewing them closed), then your intestines can slide through these holes and get stuck. This can cause an obstruction, where nothing can go through that part of your intestine. When this happens, it can cause belly pain, nausea, and vomiting. Fortunately, these are not a common occurrence, so breathe a sigh of relief!

Incisional hernias, or ventral hernias as they are called by your surgeon, occur where your surgeon made an incision in your belly. These can be small or large. What exactly are hernias? They are areas in your fascia—which is a tough tissue attached to the muscles of your abdomen, you know, like the gristle you see when you eat beef—that can weaken and form a hole. Parts of your belly can slip into the hole, for example, your intestine or fat in your belly.

If you have a small reducible hernia, then whatever stuff is sliding through the hole slides right back into your belly. We don't usually worry so much about those hernias, as long as things are sliding back into your belly. If you have a small irreducible hernia, then whatever stuff is sliding through the hole can't slide back into your belly. This can cause big problems and needs to be fixed right away.

Incisional hernias can also be large. If you've seen a large hernia, it looks like a bulge in your belly—like some alien baby is trying to get out! They're really noticeable when you try to sit up from a lying-down position. Because of the size of larger hernias, it's tough for stuff from your belly to get stuck in there, so we don't worry a lot about these.

Large hernias can cause pain or discomfort. When this happens, they can be repaired. If you choose to have your large hernia repaired, your surgeon will probably recommend that you wait until you've lost most of the weight you're going to lose. The smaller your belly is, the less pressure and tension is put on your hernia repair and the more likely it will heal without more problems. Remember, your fascia is already weakened, so any unnecessary pulling or pushing will prevent your surgeon from making a good repair.

What causes hernias to form in the first place? They can be caused by being obese, by poor nutrition (another reason to read and follow chapters 2 and 3), and by coughing a lot and coughing hard after surgery. Incisional hernias are a more common problem after surgery. So if you get one, don't panic; just make sure you tell your surgeon about it.

Anastomotic Stenosis or Stricture

The place where your stomach pouch and small intestine are stapled and sewn together can get too small or form a stenosis. This can result from inflammation, an ulcer, scar tissue, or swelling. This is something that, if it happens, may occur within weeks after surgery or years after your surgery. You may have a stenosis if you start having problems with vomiting. If you are vomiting, that means that the opening from your stomach pouch to your small intestine has narrowed so much that food can no longer pass through. The only place for the food to go is back up. To fix this, you may need to go to a gastroenterologist who will dilate the opening between your stomach and small intestine. You may need to have this area stretched more than once. If the stenosis or stricture is located where the small intestine is attached to the small intestine, then you will need to have surgery to fix this.

Malnutrition

Your small intestine has the important job of absorbing as many nutrients as it can to keep your body working well. Because part of your small intestine is bypassed during your surgery, your body has lost part of its ability to absorb nutrients. This can lead to malnutrition if you're not careful.

There are things you can do to keep this from happening. First of all, eat your protein (sound familiar?). You know from reading chapter 2 how important protein is to your body. Second of all, take your vitamins and supplements. You're going to have to swallow a lot of vitamin pills every day. You may get frustrated with doing it after a while but remember that you are eating a lot less. Your body is depending on you to take all those vitamins to keep it working well. Periodically, your doctor will have you get blood work to make sure you are not malnourished.

Ulcers

There are two kinds of ulcers that can develop after your surgery: marginal ulcers and peptic ulcers. Marginal ulcers are ulcers that can form in the area where your stomach pouch and small intestine are stapled and sewn together. The part of your small intestine that now comes off your stomach is not used to being exposed to acid from the stomach. The lining is very delicate and can develop ulcers easily. To prevent ulcers from forming, your doctor will put you on an antacid after your surgery. While having to take another pill may be annoying to you, it is important you take it. If you do develop an ulcer, some of the common symptoms you may have include chest pain or burning sensation, pain that goes through to your back, nausea, vomiting, and trouble eating.

Peptic ulcers are ulcers that can develop in your stomach pouch or in your remnant stomach (remember, your remnant stomach still makes acid). If you develop this kind of ulcer, your symptoms will be similar to the symptoms seen with a marginal ulcer.

If you smoke, you will be strongly encouraged to quit. Smoking causes irritation to the lining of your stomach (along with a laundry list of other health problems), which can lead to an ulcer. So the sooner you can quit the better.

We're making progress now! You're drinking plenty of water and fluids; you're eating right and getting your protein; you're taking all of your vitamins; you're exercising every day; your complications and other problems have been addressed. How 'bout the postsurgical blues?

DEPRESSION AND OTHER EMOTIONS

FEELING DEPRESSED ABOUT YOUR SURGERY OR WEIGHT LOSS?

Following your surgery, you may be going through a lot of emotions. You may feel happier than ever, thrilled that you went through with your surgery and excited about the results you are seeing. You may feel regret, wondering what you have done to your body, putting it through the surgery. You may feel apprehensive, wondering if your surgery will finally help you lose your weight once and for all. You may feel proud, knowing that it took a lot of courage to take this step toward better health. You may feel depressed, thinking you should be feeling better faster than you are or that you should be seeing results faster than you are.

What's causing your depression? If you are feeling depressed about the number you see when you weigh yourself, try to remember the following:

Right after your surgery, measure yourself—your arms, waist, and thighs. Then every few months measure these same areas again. Even when the number on your scale says you're not losing weight, the smaller measurements you take will show you're still doing great. You may also notice that your clothes are fitting more loosely. Remember, as you exercise, you build muscle; and muscle weighs more than fat.

Don't compare your weight loss success with that of anyone else who's had surgery—spouse, sibling or other family member, friend, or other bariatric patients. You each gained the weight differently, so you're each going to lose the weight differently. Your metabolism is not the same as everyone else's. You may be exercising more or less than everyone else. Your fluid intake may be different. Your food and caloric intake may be different. Focus on YOU and doing the best you can do.

Create a new body image of yourself. Your body image is made up of three things: the way you look at yourself in your mind's eye, the way you believe others look at you, and the way you actually feel in your own skin. Before your surgery, you probably had a poor body image. Not only did you see yourself as unattractive, but you probably felt others did too. Now that you've had your surgery and your body is changing, it's time to create your new body image.

This may take time as your new body image may not have caught up to your actual size. You may find yourself shopping for 2x, 3x, and even 4x sizes in clothing when you are only a size 16. Try standing at a full-length mirror and just look at yourself. Start at the top of your head and work down to the tips of your feet. Every time you see something you like, remember it. Remember the positive things about yourself. Are you hearing those negative things that people have said about your body in the past? Ignore them or turn them into a positive. For example, when you hear "Look at that belly!" remind yourself that it is now smaller than it was before. Keep a log of your measurements so that you have a concrete way to remind yourself of how much smaller you really are!

Next, when you think people are looking at you and thinking negative thoughts, don't try to read their minds but rather LISTEN for positive remarks and dwell on those.

And finally, the way you feel in your own skin will change as your health problems improve and your body becomes stronger. Be patient with yourself. Every now and again, look at your "before" picture, and then look at yourself now, REALLY LOOK at yourself now. Pretty different, huh? But wow, are you beautiful!

If you have a lap band and you're disappointed by your slow weight loss, remember dropping weight takes time; you should be losing about one to two pounds per week.

Since watching the number of pounds you lose each week and each month can be disappointing at times, try not to focus on your weight so much as the number of medications you no longer take. Or focus on the number of medical problems you no longer have, for example:

☺   Arthritis and joint degeneration
☺   Asthma
☺   Diabetes

☺   Enlarged heart

☺   High blood pressure

☺   High cholesterol

☺   Infertility

☺   Polycystic ovary syndrome

☺   Reflux

☺   Shortness of breath

☺   Sleep apnea

☺   Urinary incontinence

Think about how much money you're NOT spending day by day, month by month, and year by year on yourself for doctor visits, emergency room visits, medications, medical equipment (like CPAP machines, walkers, or wheelchairs), and hospitalizations.

Think of all the things you couldn't do before your surgery, which you can do now:

☺   Walk across a room without getting out of breath.

☺   Walk up and down stairs without getting out of breath or feeling pain in your knees.

☺   Sit anywhere you want at a restaurant—booth or table.

☺   Sit comfortably in an airplane—without having to ask for the seatbelt extension.

☺   Sit in movie theatre seats.

☺   Go through the turnstile at the baseball or football stadium.

☺   Get behind the wheel of your car comfortably.

☺   Get down on the floor to play with your kids or grandkids, knowing you will be able to get back up without as much trouble.

☺   Play with your kids or grandkids without getting out of breath.

☺   Ride the rollercoaster at your favorite amusement park.

☺   Shop for clothes in a regular department store.

☺   Pull up your socks and tie your shoes.

☺   Cross your legs.

☺   Find your belly button again.

☺   Sleep through the night instead of waking up gasping for air.

☺   Enjoy sex.

Think, also, of how you feel differently about yourself:

☺   More confident

☺   Proud of the new, smaller, and healthier you that is emerging

☺   Able to go out in public without fearing everyone is looking at you and judging you

☺   Able to worry less about dying too soon from obesity-related diseases

☺   Able to dream about your kids' future, knowing you
will be around to watch them grow up

☺   Happy to be photographed, not just the photographer

You may also be feeling depressed because you had
hoped that losing all your excess weight would fix the
unhappiness in your life and make your life different, but it
didn't. You still have some of the same problems you had
before your surgery. You still experience stress at home
and at work, but you have to find another way to deal
with it other than with food. Now that you have a small
stomach pouch, you can't eat like before without vomiting
or feeling chest pressure. You still experience sadness and
disappointment, but you can no longer find contentment
in food. This is called food grief. Those high-calorie sweet
foods that gave you comfort before now make you feel
miserable. You're forced to face your depression and find
a new way to deal with it or bury your feelings.

You may be feeling depressed because the one thing that
has defined you for years—your obesity—is disappearing.
Now you have to figure out who you are and who you're all
about. This can be overwhelming at times. Turn it around and
make it a time of rebirth. Before your surgery, your physical
self held you back from doing things you wanted to do. But
that isn't the case anymore. As your body becomes smaller
and healthier, you can physically do much more. Reawaken

in yourself the desire to do those things you've always wanted to do. Set your mind to it and go for it! The inner happiness that comes from motivating yourself to be all that you can will squelch the feelings of depression.

There are many other things you can do to get through your depressed feelings. First of all, talk to your doctor, physician assistant, or nurse practitioner who is caring for you. Your depression may be a result of the free-flowing estrogen in your body. Where did that come from? The fat in your body converts estrogen to a weaker form of estrogen. As you begin to lose fat, the estrogen balance is altered. And that can cause mood swings and depression. This can be corrected with hormone therapy or with time alone. Rest assured that when your weight stabilizes, so does your loss of fat and therefore the level of estrogen. If your depression is severe enough to require medical treatment and is deemed unrelated to estrogen levels, then your health care practitioner can prescribe an antidepressant for you.

Second, talk to your family. Share with them your fears, frustrations, hopes, and goals. Be careful of negative feedback, though. One of the reasons you were asked if your family supported your decision to undergo surgery was to assure that when the going became tough for you, you had some support. Be aware too that if your relationship with your spouse (kids or other family members) was already strained, don't expect your weight loss surgery to fix that relationship. Your surgery can fix your physical health problems but not your relationship problems.

If your spouse felt secure in his or her relationship with you, he or she likely won't be threatened by the looks you're getting from the opposite sex as your body becomes more attractive. If your relationship was already seeing its fair share of problems, the looks from other people may make things worse.

Your spouse may not like the physical transformation your body is going through as you lose weight. Sound strange? It's not. Your spouse may be looking at you differently, like you're a different person. Even though you know you're still the same on the inside, your spouse and those closest to you may think you're changing.

If your spouse is obese, he or she may become jealous of your new, thinner, more confident self. If you and your spouse cannot resolve the problems between you, look to a professional for help. Be prepared. Good marriages can get better; bad marriages can get worse.

Be sure to explain to your kids what's happening to you. Help them understand why you had your surgery and all the good that you hope will come from your surgery. Show them that you can physically be more involved in their lives—you can go out in public with them without them feeling embarrassed about how you look, you can play with them, and you can go to amusement parks with them and ride the scary rides with them. You are their role model from what you eat to how you prepare food, to how much you eat, to how active you are. The habits you are teaching your kids will hopefully stay with them as they get older.

Third, find support in others who have gone through what you have gone through. This can't be repeated enough; find support in others who have gone through weight loss surgery too. It's always amazing to hear one person say to another, "You felt that way too? Now I don't feel so alone. I thought I was the only one who went through that!" When someone else can empathize with you and your situation, you tend to feel better. It helps to know that someone else is going through or has gone through the same struggles as you.

Come to support group meetings whether you're five weeks, five months, five years, or fifteen years out from your surgery. The more recent your surgery, the more questions or problems you may be having that someone else can help you with. The further out from surgery you are, the more you can offer suggestions to other people. You may even learn something new that can help you!

Join an online support group. This is an anonymous way to find and offer support, which is especially good for those who feel uncomfortable talking face to face to others about such personal things.

Get the phone numbers and e-mail addresses of people who have gone through the same surgery as you. Talk to other people often! Share recipes with each other. Go to each other's homes and cook together. Go out to eat with each other. No one at the table will be giving you strange looks at the amount of food you're eating—everyone will be eating little portions! Share a ride with someone to support group meetings. Share a ride to the gym and exercise together. Share clothes with each other—you will be downsizing your wardrobe a lot, so rather than spend hundreds or thousands of dollars on new clothes, buy a few things and pass them on to a friend when you no longer fit into them.

Once again, get support by turning to those who KNOW what you're going through.

Finally, look to your friends for support. Before your surgery, some of your friends were expectedly very supportive of your decision to make yourself healthier. Others were probably questioning the safety and effectiveness of your surgery. And still others may have been flat out unsupportive, telling you that you were taking the easy way out or that the surgery was too risky to undergo.

Now that you've had your surgery, you may continue to hear the same things from the same people. It will be tough to listen to the negative comments, and you may even begin to doubt your own judgment. Try your best to ignore all that negativity. Try to help your less supportive friends understand why you had the surgery and what a difference it is making in your life. If they are still unsupportive, you may decide to exclude those people from your life altogether. Find support in those friends who are truly there for you. Focus on the good—the physical changes your body is making, the energy you are gaining, the health that you are reclaiming.

If some of your friends are overweight, they may be jealous of the success you are having. Eating may have been at the center of what you did together. Reassure these friends that you can still go out to eat but that you can't eat as much. You may want to suggest doing things together that don't involve eating. You may find that you make new friends with people who want the same things you do now. Eating may have brought you and your friends together in the past. But now, activities other than eating may bring new people, new friends, into your life.

Your coworkers can be a source of support too. You may even find that you are able to advance in your career. You are developing more energy and improved stamina, so you can now perform your job better without getting exhausted so quickly. Your boss and coworkers may feel that they can turn to you to do more. Your size and outward appearance is changing, allowing you to feel more confident. If your job requires that you be in public or give presentations, you can now do this without feeling the embarrassment you did before your surgery.

When someone in your life questions how well you are doing losing weight or someone is concerned about how little you are able to eat and worry about malnutrition, bring that person with you to your doctor's visits so that they can have their concerns addressed. Or bring that person to your support group meetings. It's reassuring to hear from other bariatric patients the ups and downs of the new lifestyle of which you are a part. The best thing you can do for yourself is to surround yourself with positive and supportive people. Remember that other people's attitudes will rub off on you. You've been given a chance at a new life; take it!

Look at you go! You're drinking plenty of water and fluids; you're eating right and getting your protein; you're taking all of your vitamins; you're exercising every day; your complications and other problems have been addressed; you're curing the blues. Let's talk recipes.

RECIPES

NEED RECIPE OR QUICK-MEAL IDEAS?

You now know how important it is for you to drink enough water and other fluids, eat adequate servings of protein, and get your vitamins and nutrients. But now you're thinking, *I need ideas!* You're tired of eating chili every day. If you look at one more chicken breast, you're going to get "clucking" mad.

There are only so many ways to prepare chicken, turkey, pork, ham, eggs, and fish; actually, there are MANY ways to prepare chicken, turkey, pork, ham, eggs, and fish. You can use different spices to give your meat or fish different flavors. You can bake, broil, or grill your meat or fish. You can hard-boil eggs or scramble them or poach them or try them sunny-side up or over easy. Or you can make an omelet using ingredients like turkey, ham, bacon, peppers, peanut butter (hey don't knock it 'til you've tried it—it's yummy!), or cheese. Try tofu for a change of pace. Tofu is bland by itself, but it will take on the flavor of whatever spices you cook it in. Just think how many different combinations of spices there are—Chinese, Indian, Italian, Mexican, Polish—and the list goes on.

You can bake or steam some vegetables to go with your protein. Or you can couple your protein with a salad. Use your imagination!

If you're still stumped and need ideas, ask your spouse or kids what sounds good to them. Call a friend and ask him or her for suggestions. You may think that because you can only eat small meals that you are limited in what you can eat. But you're not. Your diet can be just as varied as it was before your surgery. Just be sure to eat your proteins first and carbohydrates second.

One of the most basic food items you will probably come back to over and over again is your protein shake. There are many ways to make protein shakes, and you may even choose to buy them already made. The following shake recipe is very simple and gives you about fifty grams of protein in about eight ounces of fluid. This is an especially good recipe to use early after your surgery when you feel the most restricted. With only a little bit of fluid you can get a lot of protein. Here's the recipe:

(Adapted from *Before and After: Living & Eating Well After Weight loss Surgery* by Susan Maria Leach)

Protein Shakes—Twenty-one Variations

Basic Shake Recipe
½ cup skim milk, soy milk, or water
2 scoops vanilla protein powder*
1 cup ice cubes
Flavoring ingredients (optional, see below)**

*choose protein powder containing twenty to thirty grams of protein per scoop and low carbohydrates

Measure the ingredients into a blender. Pulse the blender on and off until the ingredients are well blended and creamy. You don't need to add more liquid to the shake. Do not turn the blender on and leave it on the high setting. This will make your shake dense and foamy. You will be drinking a lot of air volume, which can make you feel uncomfortable.

**Optional flavoring ingredients:
Frozen banana chunk—cut a ripe banana into two-inch pieces, wrap each piece individually in plastic wrap, and freeze

Frozen papaya or mango cubes—peel and seed a ripe papaya or mango, cut it into two-inch cubes, wrap each piece individually in plastic wrap, and freeze

Frozen pineapple cubes—in an ice cube tray, place about one tablespoon of crushed pineapple and juice into each section and freeze

Try any one of the following and go bananas!
- ☺   1 banana chunk and 1 teaspoon maple extract
- ☺   1 banana chunk and ¼ teaspoon cinnamon and ½ teaspoon vanilla extract
- ☺   1 banana chunk and 1/8 teaspoon freshly grated nutmeg and ½ teaspoon vanilla extract

☺   1 banana chunk and ¼ cup orange juice and ½ teaspoon vanilla extract and replace milk (in basic recipe) with ¼ cup water

☺   1 banana chunk and 2 teaspoons cocoa powder and ½ teaspoon vanilla extract

☺   1 banana chunk and 2 tablespoons sugar-free hazelnut syrup

☺   1 banana chunk and 1 heaping tablespoon whipped peanut butter and ½ teaspoon vanilla extract

For a more fruity drink, try any one of these:

☺   2 papaya cubes and 1 banana chunk and 1 teaspoon coconut extract and ½ teaspoon vanilla extract

☺   2 pineapple cubes and ½ teaspoon coconut extract and ½ teaspoon vanilla extract

☺   1 pineapple cube and 3 frozen strawberries and ½ teaspoon vanilla extract

These may remind you more of dessert or an after dinner coffee treat:

☺   ¼ cup frozen cherries and ½ teaspoon almond extract and ½ teaspoon vanilla extract

☺   2 sugar-free chocolate cream-filled sandwich cookies and 1 heaping tablespoon Cool Whip and ½ teaspoon vanilla extract

☺   2 teaspoons cocoa powder and ½ teaspoon vanilla extract and ¼ teaspoon cinnamon

☺   ¼ cup no-sugar-added applesauce and ½ teaspoon cinnamon and 1 tablespoon sugar-free hazelnut syrup

☺   2 teaspoons cocoa powder and 1 heaping tablespoon whipped peanut butter and ½ teaspoon vanilla extract

☺   2 teaspoons cocoa powder and ¼ cup frozen cherries and ½ teaspoon almond extract

☺   2 teaspoons cocoa powder and 1 teaspoon coconut extract and ½ teaspoon vanilla extract

☺   ½ teaspoon instant espresso and 2 teaspoons cocoa powder and ½ teaspoon vanilla extract

☺   1 teaspoon instant espresso and 2 tablespoons sugar-free hazelnut syrup and pinch of cinnamon

☺   1 teaspoon instant espresso and ¼ teaspoon cinnamon

If you had the lap band procedure, you will also be asked to maintain a pureed diet for a couple weeks after your surgery. You will likely need a food processor to puree your food. You can use a blender too, but you may find that the food processor works better. Here are some tips to follow to prepare your food more easily:

☺ Make sure the food you cook comes out as soft and moist as possible—a Crock Pot is great for this.

☺ Cut the food into small pieces before putting it into the food processor.

☺ Slowly add liquid to the food processor to reach the consistency you want.

☺ Food will puree best when it is still warm or hot.

☺ Foods with nuts, seeds, skins, or stringy foods do not puree as well.

☺ When you puree fish, try adding lemon juice, mayonnaise, or tartar sauce.

☺ Meats (like chicken, beef, pork, or turkey) can be pureed using sauces, broth, or gravy.

☺ If you want to eat your vegetables, steam them first then puree them.

☺ You can puree pasta or rice—just be sure it is very tender.

☺ Chunky soups or chili can be pureed.

☺ Chicken salad, tuna salad, or egg salad can be pureed.

☺ When in doubt, buy baby food—the pureeing is done for you!

As you become accustomed to your new lifestyle and learn how to eat, you will probably find that it is hard to prepare just ONE meal at a time—you will likely be preparing food that will be enough for many meals. Face it; you fix a pot of chili; you're eating chili for a week. So pick recipes that you really like and buy SMALL food containers for storing each of your portions and be prepared to see the same meal again and again. If you don't already have a Crock Pot, you might want to get one as you can prepare enough food for yourself for a week all at one time.

Can't stand the thought of eating chili for the next seven days? Get a group of five or six "bariatric buddies" together, and fix five or six different dishes and share them. Each of you can take home small food containers with each of the different home-cooked meals and enjoy a different one every day. Or if you have the time yourself, fix two to three different meals on the weekend, divide them up into small servings, and then over the course of the next couple weeks rotate what meal you eat. Get creative!

You're undoubtedly thinking, *I wish I could find small meals already prepared. Then all I have to do is toss one in the microwave and be done with it*. Well, you can. Check out the freezer section of your favorite grocery store. Many of the frozen dinners will be too big for just one meal, but there are some that are a more appropriate size. Healthy Choice, Smart Ones, Kashi, Lean Cuisine, and Michelina's Lean Gourmet meals average nine to ten ounces per serving. Try to stay away from the meals that are mostly pasta. You should be eating mostly protein and only some carbohydrates.

If you like pita pockets for making sandwiches using tuna or chicken salad (or ham salad, or egg salad, or . . .), you can find mini pita pockets in both original and wheat at Trader Joe's.

As the holidays roll around, you may be wondering if you will be able to enjoy some of your favorite holiday dishes. You may have to substitute more unhealthy ingredients for healthier ones (like using Stevia or Truvia instead of sugar), but you can still indulge. Always remember to get your protein in first (where have I heard this?). Avoid high fat and sweet foods as much as possible. If you can only eat a small spoonful of mashed potatoes or green bean casserole with your turkey, that's okay. Sometimes all you need is a taste of your favorite food. Then you're satisfied until the next holiday! The following recipe is a great one for Thanksgiving or Christmas or any time you feel like pumpkin pie:

Pumpkin Fluff Dip
Ingredients:
1 15 oz can of Pumpkin
1 6 oz box of Sugar-free Instant Vanilla Pudding
1 16 oz tub of Cool Whip*

Combine the pumpkin with instant vanilla pudding and mix well. Then fold in the Cool Whip. This can be served with cinnamon graham crackers, bananas, or apples. Refrigerate any unused portion.

(Marlene E.—bariatric patient)

*If you want to increase the amount of protein in this recipe, add ricotta cheese instead of Cool Whip.

The following are main dish recipes that are available at RealSimple.com. This Web site offers MANY different recipes, and this is just a small sampling of them. Feel free to reduce or eliminate the amount of salt in these recipes to decrease the total sodium content. You will notice that listed in parentheses are the calories, fat grams, saturated fat grams, polyunsaturated fat grams (poly fat), monounsaturated fat grams (mono fat), calcium, cholesterol, carbohydrates, sodium, protein, fiber, and sugar content.

Beef

Southwestern Beef Chili with Corn

1 tablespoon olive oil

2 carrots, chopped

1 medium onion, chopped

1 poblano or bell pepper, chopped

½ pound ground beef

2 tablespoons tomato paste

2 15-ounce cans black beans, drained and rinsed

1 tablespoon chili powder

Kosher salt and pepper

½ cup corn kernels (from 1 ear, or frozen and thawed)

½ cup grated cheddar (2 ounces)

2 scallions, sliced

Heat the oil in a large saucepan over medium-high heat. Add the carrots, onion, and poblano and cook, stirring, for three minutes.

Add the beef and cook, breaking it up with a spoon, until it is no longer pink, three to five minutes.

Add the tomato paste and cook, stirring, until it is slightly darkened, one minute. Add the beans, chili powder, three cups water, one-half teaspoon salt, and one-fourth teaspoon pepper. Simmer over medium heat until the vegetables are tender, about ten minutes.

Stir in the corn. Divide among bowls and top with the cheddar and scallions.

Make ahead: You can cook the chili in advance and refrigerate it for up to three days or freeze it for up to three months.

(Calories 343; fat 15g; sat. fat 5g; cholesterol 51mg; carbohydrates 34g; sodium 893mg; protein 23g; fiber 11g; sugar 6g)

Sara Quessenberry, Real Simple, September 2008

Chicken

Asian Chicken with Brussels Sprouts

1/3 cup low-sodium soy sauce

1/3 cup rice vinegar

¼ cup dark brown sugar

2 tablespoons grated ginger

2 cups low-sodium chicken broth

1 ½ pounds boneless, skinless chicken breast, cut into 1-inch pieces

2 carrots, cut into 1/8-inch rounds

8 ounces brussels sprouts, thinly sliced or shredded

2 scallions (white and light green parts), sliced

Combine the soy sauce, vinegar, sugar, ginger, and chicken broth in a medium saucepan and bring to a boil. Add the chicken and carrots and simmer for six minutes.

Stir in the brussels sprouts and continue cooking until the chicken is cooked through, about two minutes more. Divide among individual bowls and top with the scallions.

Upgrade: Add more flavor to this dish by drizzling it with aromatic toasted sesame oil just before serving.

(Calories 246; fat 3g; sat. fat 0g; cholesterol 66mg; carbohydrates 21g; sodium 843mg; protein 32g; fiber 4g; sugar 4g)

Sara Quessenberry, Real Simple, November 2007

Chicken and Bok Choy Stir-Fry

1 tablespoon canola oil

4 6-ounce boneless, skinless chicken breasts, cut into 1-inch pieces

Kosher salt and black pepper

4 heads baby bok choy, quartered lengthwise

¼ cup low-sodium soy sauce

¼ cup store-bought barbecue sauce

4 scallions, thinly sliced

Heat the oil in a large skillet over medium-high heat.

Season the chicken with one-fourth teaspoon each salt and pepper and cook, tossing occasionally, until browned and cooked through, four to six minutes. Transfer to a plate.

Add the bok choy and one-fourth cup water to the skillet. Cover and cook until the bok choy is just tender, three to four minutes.

In a small bowl, combine the soy sauce, barbecue sauce, and scallions. Add to the skillet and bring to a boil. Return the chicken to the skillet and cook, tossing, until heated through, one to two minutes.

(Calories 268; fat 8g, sat. fat 1g; cholesterol 94mg; carbohydrates 11g; sodium 837mg; protein 37g; fiber 2g; sugar 6g)

Kate Merker and Sara Quessenberry,
Real Simple, October 2008

Chicken Sautéed with Apples

4 boneless, skinless chicken-breast halves
1 tablespoon olive oil
1 firm apple, such as Braeburn, cored, halved, and cut into ½ inch slices
1 cup apple juice
1 large onion, thinly sliced
1 garlic clove, minced
½ teaspoon dried thyme leaves
½ teaspoon salt
2 tablespoons Dijon mustard

Place each chicken-breast half between two sheets of wax paper and pound with a meat mallet until about three-fourth inch thick.

Heat the oil in a large skillet over medium-high heat and sauté the chicken until golden, about three minutes per side.

Add the apple slices, apple juice, onion, garlic, thyme, and salt. Cover and simmer six to eight minutes or until the chicken is fork-tender. Remove the chicken, apple slices, and onion to a serving platter and keep warm.

Bring the sauce to a boil for about five minutes or until slightly reduced. Whisk in the mustard. Pour the sauce over the chicken and serve.

(Calories 255.7; fat 7.52g, sat. fat 1.45g; cholesterol 78.31mg; calcium 43.96mg; carbohydrates 17g; sodium 551.89mg; protein 29.61g; fiber 1.59g; iron 1.76mg)

Jane Kirby and Kay Chun, Real Simple,
October 2002

Coconut Chicken

4 boneless, skinless chicken breast halves

1 tablespoon olive oil

2 garlic cloves, peeled and cut in half lengthwise

¼ teaspoon crushed red pepper flakes or 1 sliced small red Thai chili

1 teaspoon kosher salt

Freshly ground black pepper

1 (14-ounce) can light coconut milk

Shredded zest and juice of 1 lime

1 tablespoon Thai fish sauce

2 tablespoons cilantro leaves, chopped

Using a rolling pin, pound the chicken between two sheets of wax paper until they are of uniform thickness.

Heat the oil, garlic, and red pepper flakes in a large skillet over medium-high heat until the oil shimmers and the garlic browns. (Don't burn the garlic.) Add the chicken breasts and cook until golden, three to five minutes on each side.

Add the salt, pepper, coconut milk, and lime zest and juice. Cover, reduce heat to medium-low, and cook three minutes longer or until the chicken is fork-tender.

Remove the chicken to a platter and keep warm. Increase heat to high and boil the sauce until thickened or syrupy, three to five minutes. Whisk in the fish sauce and pour the sauce over the chicken. Garnish with cilantro.

(Calories 252; fat 13g; sat. fat 8g; cholesterol 78mg; calcium 53mg; carbohydrates 4g; sodium 992mg; protein 29g; fiber 0g; iron 1mg)

Jane Kirby, Real Simple, February 2003

Crunchy Herbed Chicken

4 slices white bread, toasted

½ cup fresh flat-leaf parsley

1 clove garlic, chopped

Kosher salt and black pepper

1 tablespoon olive oil

¼ cup Dijon mustard

4 6-ounce boneless, skinless chicken breasts

Heat oven to 400°F.

In a food processor, pulse the bread, parsley, garlic, and one-fourth teaspoon each of salt and pepper until coarse crumbs form. Add the oil and pulse to combine. Transfer to a plate.

Spread the mustard over the chicken and dip the pieces in the bread-crumb mixture, pressing gently to help it adhere. Place on a baking sheet and bake until golden and cooked through, eighteen to twenty minutes.

(Calories 286; fat 8g, sat. fat 2g; cholesterol 94mg; carbohydrates 14g; sodium 456mg; protein 37g; fiber 1g; sugar 2g)

Kate Merker and Sara Quessenberry,

Real Simple, October 2008

Feta Chicken with Zucchini

2 tablespoons olive oil

1 lemon

4 boneless, skinless chicken breasts (about 1 ½ pounds)

¼ teaspoon kosher salt

2 medium zucchini

¼ cup fresh flat-leaf parsley leaves, chopped

1/8 teaspoon black pepper

1/3 cup (about 2 ounces) crumbled Feta

Heat oven to 400°F.

Drizzle one-half tablespoon of the oil in a roasting pan. Remove the zest from the lemon in thin strips; set aside.

Thinly slice the lemon. Place half the slices in the pan. Rinse the chicken and pat it dry with paper towels. Place it on top of the lemon slices and season with one-eighth teaspoon of the salt.

Slice each zucchini in half lengthwise then slice each half into one-fourth-inch-thick half-moons. In a bowl, combine the zucchini, parsley, pepper, and the remaining oil, lemon slices, and salt; toss. Spread the zucchini mixture around the chicken and sprinkle the Feta over the top. Roast until the chicken is cooked through, twenty to twenty-five minutes.

Transfer it to a cutting board and cut each piece into thirds. Divide the chicken, zucchini mixture, and lemons among individual plates and sprinkle with the zest.

(Calories 270; fat 8g, sat. fat 3g; cholesterol 110mg; carbohydrates 5g; sodium 378mg; protein 42g; fiber 2g; sugar 3g)

Real Simple, June 2006

Hoisin-Glazed Chicken with Cabbage Slaw

4 boneless, skinless chicken cutlets

1/3 cup hoisin sauce

1 tablespoon low-sodium soy sauce

1 tablespoon plus 1 teaspoon rice vinegar

2 teaspoons fish sauce (optional)

3 cups shredded green cabbage

1 red bell pepper, cut into strips

1 green bell pepper, cut into strips

3 scallions, halved and cut into 4-inch strips

½ cup fresh cilantro leaves

Heat broiler on high.

Rinse the cutlets and pat dry with paper towels. Pound the cutlets to an even thinness. Place on a broiler pan.

In a small bowl, whisk together the hoisin sauce, soy sauce, one teaspoon of the rice vinegar, and the fish sauce (if using).

Transfer two tablespoons of the glaze to a large bowl and stir in the remaining rice vinegar. Add the cabbage, peppers, scallions, and cilantro and toss. Cover and refrigerate.

Pour about one tablespoon of the remaining glaze into a small bowl; set aside as a finishing sauce. Brush the chicken with the glaze that remains. Broil, brushing occasionally, until cooked through, five to eight minutes.

Spoon the reserved glaze over the top. Serve with the slaw.

(Calories 272; fat 3g, sat. fat 0.7g, poly fat 0.9g, mono fat 0.8g; carbohydrates 16g; protein 44g; fiber 3g; sugar 5g)

Real Simple, February 2006

Fish

Asian-Style Halibut in Parchment

1 small head bok choy, thickly sliced, or 4 baby bok choy, ends trimmed

1 red bell pepper, thinly sliced lengthwise

4 6-ounce halibut fillets

½ teaspoon black pepper

3 scallions (white and green parts), thinly sliced on a diagonal

Zest from ½ orange, cut into matchstick-size strips

3 tablespoons low-sodium soy sauce

1 ½ teaspoons rice vinegar

1 ½ teaspoons sesame oil

2 teaspoons grated ginger root

Heat oven to 400°F.

Tear off four fifteen-inch squares of parchment paper or aluminum foil and arrange on two baking sheets. Divide the bok choy and bell pepper evenly among the squares. Place a halibut fillet on each mound of vegetables and sprinkle with the black pepper. Top with the scallions and zest.

In a small bowl, combine the soy sauce, vinegar, oil, and ginger. Spoon the mixture evenly over the halibut. Top with four more squares of parchment or foil and fold the edges over several times to seal. Bake for fifteen minutes.

Transfer each packet to a plate. Serve with a knife to slit the package open, and be careful of the steam that will escape.

Tip: This beautiful meal works just as well with other types of seafood. Next time, try cod, salmon, sea scallops, or peeled and deveined shrimp.

(Calories 231; fat 6g, sat. fat 1g; cholesterol 54mg; carbohydrates 5g; sodium 524mg; protein 38g; fiber 1g; sugar 4g)

Kate Merker, Real Simple,

December 2006

Cedar-Plank Salmon

Cedar boards for grilling are sold at gourmet food shops, houseware stores, and lumberyards. (Make sure the lumber hasn't been treated with preservatives or other chemicals.) The fish comes out smoky and moist. You'll never grill salmon the traditional way again.

1 2-pound salmon fillet, skin on
1 cedar plank, soaked in water 20 minutes
½ cup brown sugar
2 tablespoons canola oil
1 tablespoon dried thyme leaves
1 teaspoon cayenne pepper

Preheat a gas grill to high; adjust to medium low after fifteen minutes. (If cooking over charcoal, allow the coals to burn until they are covered with white ash.) Place the salmon skin-side down on the cedar plank.

Combine the brown sugar, oil, thyme, and cayenne in a bowl. Spread over the salmon. Place the planked salmon on the grilling grate and cook, with grill covered, about forty minutes or just until the surface fat begins to turn white.

Rainy-day Method: Preheat oven to 325°F. Prepare the salmon as described above then roast on the cedar plank for about twenty-five minutes.

(Calories 550; fat 32g, sat. fat 5g; cholesterol 134mg; calcium 63mg; carbohydrates 19g; sodium 142mg; protein 45g; fiber 1g; iron 3mg)

Jane Kirby, Real Simple, June 2003

Chili-rubbed Salmon

1 ½ tablespoons chili powder

½ teaspoon dried oregano

¼ teaspoon kosher salt

1 ½ pounds skinless salmon fillet (4 pieces), 4 skinless, boneless chicken-breast halves, or 2 pork tenderloins, halved (1 ½ to 2 pounds total)

1 tablespoon olive oil

In a bowl, combine the chili powder, oregano, and salt. Pat the spices on the fish or meat.

Heat the oil in a large nonstick skillet over medium heat. Cook five minutes per side for the salmon, eight to ten minutes per side for the chicken, or fifteen minutes per side for the pork. (Reduce the heat if the spices begin to turn black.)

Divide the fish or meat among four plates.

(Calories 351; fat 22g, sat. fat 4g; cholesterol 100mg; calcium 32mg; carbohydrates 2g; sodium 274mg; protein 34g; fiber 1g; iron 1mg)

Jane Kirby and Leslie Pendleton, Real Simple, April 2004

Grilled Mahi-mahi with Grapefruit, Avocado, and Watercress Salad

4 6-ounce pieces mahi-mahi, skin removed

1 teaspoon plus 2 tablespoons extra-virgin olive oil

Kosher salt and pepper

1 grapefruit

2 tablespoons fresh lime juice

2 teaspoons honey

2 scallions, trimmed and thinly sliced

2 bunches watercress, thick stems removed

1 avocado, cut into chunks

Heat a grill, or grill pan to medium-high.

Rub the mahi-mahi with one teaspoon of the oil and season with one-fourth teaspoon salt and one-eighth teaspoon pepper. Grill until cooked through and opaque, about five minutes per side, depending on the thickness.

Meanwhile, cut away the peel and white pith of the grapefruit with a knife and slice the fruit into one-fourth-inch rounds.

In a small bowl, combine the remaining oil, lime juice, honey, one-half teaspoon salt, one-eighth teaspoon pepper, and scallions.

Divide the watercress, avocado, and grapefruit among individual plates. Place the mahi-mahi on top and drizzle with the lime dressing.

(Calories 315; fat 14g, sat. fat 2g; cholesterol 125mg; carbohydrates 14g; sodium 405mg; protein 33g; fiber 3g; sugar 12g)

Sara Quessenberry, Real Simple, March 2008

Pan-roasted Salmon and White Beans

1 ½ pounds salmon steaks, about ¾ inch thick

2 tablespoons all-purpose flour

2 tablespoons olive oil

½ teaspoon kosher salt

Freshly ground black pepper

1 14 1/2-ounce can diced tomatoes

1 16-ounce can small white navy beans (drained)

2 garlic cloves, minced

2 tablespoons chopped fresh tarragon

Dredge the fish in the flour.

Meanwhile, heat the oil in a large skillet over medium heat until it shimmers. Add the fish and brown about three minutes on each side. Carefully lift the fish out of the skillet and set it aside on a platter; sprinkle with the salt and pepper.

Add the tomatoes, beans, and garlic to the skillet and bring to a boil over high heat. Cook three minutes.

Reduce heat to low, return the fish to the pan and add tarragon. Cover and cook five minutes or until the fish flakes when tested with a fork or the tip of a knife.

(Calories 505; fat 26g, sat. fat 5g; cholesterol 100mg; calcium 142mg; carbohydrates 27g; sodium 673mg; protein 41g; fiber 4g; iron 3mg)

Jane Kirby, Real Simple, February 2003

Roasted Fennel and Red Onion Salmon

2 small fennel bulbs, cut into 1/2-inch wedges

1 large red onion, cut into 1/2-inch wedges

6 cloves garlic, smashed

1 cup cherry or grape tomatoes

2 teaspoons extra-virgin olive oil

½ bunch fresh thyme sprigs

1 teaspoon kosher salt

½ teaspoon freshly ground black pepper

4 6-ounce salmon fillets, skinned

1 lemon, halved

Heat oven to 400°F.

In a roasting pan, toss the fennel, onion, garlic, tomatoes, thyme, one-half teaspoon of the salt, one-fourth teaspoon of the pepper, and the oil. Spread evenly and roast for twenty minutes.

Move the vegetables to side of pan, add the salmon, then redistribute the vegetables around the salmon. Squeeze the lemon halves over the salmon. Sprinkle the salmon with the remaining salt and pepper.

Return to oven and roast until the salmon is the same color throughout and flakes easily, ten to twelve minutes. Serve immediately.

Tip: When estimating how long to cook fish, allow about ten minutes for each inch of thickness.

(Calories 394.71; fat 21.08g, sat. fat 4.06g; cholesterol 100.36mg; calcium 99.87mg; carbohydrates 15.19g; sodium 430.36mg; protein 36.17g; fiber 4.4g; iron 2.21mg)

Kate Merker, Real Simple, October 2005

Salmon with Black Bean Sauce

2 tablespoons soy sauce

2 teaspoons sugar

½ cup canola oil

2 teaspoons cornstarch

1 ½ cups canned chicken stock

4 6-ounce salmon fillets (1 inch thick)

2 garlic cloves, minced

1 tablespoon peeled, minced fresh ginger

2 tablespoons jarred black bean sauce (available in the Asian section of most supermarkets)

2 teaspoons rice or white wine vinegar

¼ cup grated carrots

¼ cup grated radishes

¼ cup slivered scallions

In a large bowl, combine the soy sauce, sugar, and one-fourth cup of the oil. In a small bowl, combine the cornstarch and chicken stock. Set both aside.

Make three slashes on the skin side of each salmon fillet, cutting halfway into the fish. Place the salmon in a shallow dish and pour the soy-sauce marinade over it. Refrigerate for thirty minutes.

In a medium saucepan, heat the remaining one-fourth cup of oil over medium heat and add the garlic, ginger, and black bean sauce. Cook for one to two minutes or until the garlic is golden. Add the vinegar and the cornstarch mixture. Bring to a boil then reduce to a simmer. Cook for ten minutes, remove from heat, and keep warm.

Remove the fish from the marinade and place on a foil-lined broiler pan, about three inches from the heat. Broil three to four minutes per side until just cooked through (center should be slightly translucent). Serve the salmon topped with the sauce and the raw vegetables.

(Calories 609; fat 47g, sat. fat 6g; cholesterol 100mg; calcium 39mg; carbohydrates 8g; sodium 691mg; protein 37g; fiber 1g; iron 1mg)

Rori Spinelli-Trovato, Real Simple,

March 2001

Salmon with Dijon Dill Sauce

4 6-ounce salmon fillets, skin removed

½ teaspoon kosher salt

1 tablespoon olive oil

3 tablespoons unsalted butter, cold

1 small shallot, finely chopped

½ cup white wine

1 tablespoon Dijon mustard

2 tablespoons roughly chopped fresh dill, plus more for garnishing

1/8 teaspoon black pepper

1 cucumber, thinly sliced (optional)

Set broiler on high. Place the salmon on a foil-lined broiler pan and season with one-fourth teaspoon of the salt. Broil until the salmon is the same color throughout and flakes easily, seven to ten minutes, depending on thickness.

Meanwhile, in a medium saucepan, over medium-high heat, heat the oil and one tablespoon of the butter until it melts. Add the shallot and cook until softened, about one minute. Add the wine and cook until reduced by half, about three minutes.

Reduce heat to low and whisk in the mustard, dill, pepper, and the remaining salt. Remove from heat.

Cut the remaining butter into pieces, add to the sauce, and whisk until incorporated. Place the salmon on individual plates, spoon the sauce over the top, and sprinkle with additional dill. Serve with the cucumber (if desired).

Tara Bench, Real Simple, September 2006

Scallops in Parchment
1 pint cherry or grape tomatoes
1 15-ounce can white beans, rinsed
1 fennel bulb, halved, cored, and thinly sliced
½ cup fresh flat-leaf parsley leaves, chopped
2 teaspoons extra-virgin olive oil
½ teaspoon kosher salt
¼ teaspoon black pepper
1 ½ pounds sea scallops, rinsed and patted dry

Heat oven to 400°F.

Gently toss the tomatoes, beans, fennel, parsley, oil, salt, and pepper in a large bowl.

Tear off four fifteen-inch squares of parchment paper and arrange on two baking sheets. Spoon some of the bean mixture into the center of each square. Place the scallops on top of the beans. Top with four more squares of parchment and fold the edges over several times to seal. Bake for fifteen minutes.

Transfer each packet to a plate. Serve with a knife to slit the package open, and be careful of the steam that will escape.

(Calories 339; fat 4g, sat. fat 0.5g, poly fat 1.0g, mono fat 1.8g; carbohydrates 37g; protein 39g; fiber 9g; sugar 3.5g)

Real Simple, February 2006

Spice-Baked Sea Bass and Red Lentils
3 tablespoons olive oil
1 large yellow onion, finely chopped
2 cloves garlic, finely chopped
2 teaspoons ground ginger
1 ½ teaspoons ground cumin
16 ounces red or green lentils, washed and drained
4 cups low-sodium chicken or vegetable broth
3 tablespoons fresh lemon juice
½ teaspoon black pepper
1 ¼ teaspoons kosher salt
½ teaspoon ground coriander (optional)
½ teaspoon dried thyme
4 6-ounce sea bass fillets, skin removed

Heat oven to 400°F.

Heat two tablespoons of the oil in a large saucepan over medium heat. Add the onion and cook for seven minutes or until soft. Add the garlic, ginger, and cumin and cook, stirring, for one minute. Add the lentils and broth and bring to a boil. Reduce heat and simmer, stirring occasionally, until the lentils are tender, about twenty minutes.

Stir in the lemon juice, one-fourth teaspoon of the pepper, and three-fourth teaspoon of the salt. Remove from heat.

Meanwhile, in a small bowl, combine the coriander (if using), thyme, and the remaining salt and pepper. Place the fish in a baking dish, drizzle with the remaining oil, and sprinkle the tops with the spice mixture. Bake until the fish is the same color throughout and flakes easily, about ten minutes.

Divide the lentils among individual plates and serve with the fish.

Tip: If sea bass isn't available, you can substitute another firm fish, such as grouper, cod, or halibut.

(Calories 443; fat 16g, sat. fat 1g; cholesterol 70mg; carbohydrates 34g; sodium 791mg; protein 47g; fiber 1g; sugar 8g)

Kate Merker, Real Simple, May 2007

Steamed Fish and Vegetables

1 head broccoli, cut into florets

3 yellow squash or zucchini, cut into 1/2-inch rounds

¾ teaspoon kosher salt

4 8-ounce skinless halibut fillets (about 1 inch thick)

¼ teaspoon black pepper

4 teaspoons extra-virgin olive oil

2 tablespoons finely chopped fresh herbs (such as basil, flat-leaf parsley, or thyme) (optional)

2 lemons, halved

Place a steamer in a large saucepan. Add enough water to reach just below it. Bring to a boil. Add the vegetables, cover, and steam until tender, about seven minutes. Transfer to a bowl and season with one-fourth teaspoon of the salt. Cover to keep warm.

If necessary, add more water to the pan. Return to a boil. Season the halibut with the remaining salt and the pepper. Place the halibut on the steamer, cover, and cook until it flakes easily and is the same color throughout, about seven minutes.

Drizzle the halibut and vegetables with the oil. Sprinkle with the herbs (if using) and serve the lemon halves on the side.

(Calories 295; fat 9g, sat. fat 1.3g, poly fat 1.9g, mono fat 4.6g; carbohydrates 17g; protein 40g; fiber 7g; sugar 6g)

Real Simple, February 2006

Vegetarian

Chickpea Pasta with Almonds and Parmesan

1 tablespoon olive oil

3 cloves garlic, chopped

7 cups low-sodium vegetable or chicken broth

½ teaspoon crushed red pepper flakes

Kosher salt

1 pound angel hair pasta

1 15.5-ounce can chickpeas, drained and rinsed

1 cup flat-leaf parsley, chopped

¼ cup unsalted roasted almonds, chopped

½ cup grated Parmesan

Heat the oil in a large saucepan over medium-high heat. Stir in the garlic and cook for one minute. Add the broth, red pepper, and three-fourth teaspoon salt and bring to a boil.

Add the pasta and cook, stirring, until the broth is nearly absorbed and the pasta is al dente, about six minutes. Stir in the chickpeas and parsley.

Divide among individual bowls and top with the almonds and parmesan.

(Calories 652; fat 14g, sat. fat 1g; cholesterol 8mg; carbohydrates 110g; sodium 782mg; protein 26g; fiber 7g; sugar 6g)

Sara Quessenberry, Real Simple, January 2008

Vegetable Chili with Polenta

3 tablespoons olive oil

1 large onion, finely chopped

2 garlic cloves, minced

2 tablespoons chili powder

1 ½ teaspoons ground cumin

1 14.5-ounce can diced tomatoes with juice

1 15.5-ounce can red kidney beans, rinsed and drained

1 15.5-ounce can cannellini or great northern beans, rinsed and drained

1 8-ounce can vegetarian beans (or pork and beans)

1 tablespoon red wine vinegar

½ cup quick-cooking polenta

1 tablespoon butter

Green chili or jalapeño salsa, optional

Heat the oil in a large skillet over medium heat. Add the onion, garlic, chili powder, and cumin and sauté until onions are soft. Add the tomatoes and 1 cup of water. Bring to a simmer, partially cover with a lid, and cook for ten minutes.

Add the beans and return to a simmer; continue cooking, uncovered, twenty minutes, until the chili is thick.

Remove from heat and stir in the vinegar. Season to taste with salt and freshly ground pepper.

While the chili cooks, prepare the polenta according to package directions (five to eight minutes) and stir in the butter. Season to taste with salt and freshly ground pepper. Divide between four bowls and ladle chili over top. Spoon a little salsa on top, if desired.

(Calories 468; fat 15g, sat. fat 3g; cholesterol 8mg; calcium 190mg; carbohydrates 72g; sodium 770mg; protein 17g; fiber 14g; iron 6mg)

Susan Quick, Real Simple, May 2000

Still can't think of anything that sounds good to eat? Are you still incredibly bored with your current menu? When you, your family, and your friends are stumped on what to try next, try a recipe book. While just about any recipe book can offer you the variety for which you're looking—whether it's Chinese, French, German, Indian, Italian, Japanese, Mexican, Polish, Puerto Rican, Vietnamese, or ("whew!") American food—you may be interested in recipes designed specifically for bariatric patients. The following books contain various recipes geared toward people who have undergone bariatric surgery:

☺   *Before and After Living & Eating Well After Weight Loss Surgery* by Susan Maria Leach contains one hundred different recipe ideas

☺   *Eating Well After Weight Loss Surgery* by Patt Levine, Michele Bontmpo-Saray, William B. Inabnet—for those who had the lap band procedure

☺   *Extraordinary Taste: A Festive Guide for Life After Weight Loss Surgery* by Shannon Owens-Malett

☺   *Recipes for Life After Weight loss Surgery: Delicious Dishes for Nourishing the New You* by Margaret Furtado and Lynette Schultz

The Internet can also be a source of recipe ideas specifically for bariatric patients. BariatricEating.com has great recipes!

We're almost there! You're drinking plenty of water and fluids; you're eating right and getting your protein; you're taking all of your vitamins; you're exercising every day; your complications and other problems have been addressed; you're curing the blues; you've got more recipes than you can shake a spoon at. Let's look into the future.

MOVING FORWARD

WHERE WILL YOU GO FROM HERE?

Never Obese Again

When you look into the future and picture yourself, do you see yourself as the thinner, healthier, happier person you wanted to be? Can you picture the new you? Is the future a blur to you—you're not sure if you will lose your weight once and for all or if you will gain it back AGAIN. One way to be successful is to see yourself as successful.

It may be hard to believe that you can actually lose your weight this time and never go back to being obese. You've tried so many different diets, and none of them worked. Why should surgery work? Surgery is the powerful tool that lets you feel full—maybe for the first time in your life. Surgery is the powerful tool that limits the volume of food you can eat. The rest is up to you. You have to choose what kind of food you're going to eat. You have to choose to drink enough fluids. You have to choose to take your vitamins. You have to choose to exercise. You have to choose to change your way of living to not only take the weight off but keep it off. You have to change your way of living to make your health problems that came with obesity go away and stay away.

It is very important that you follow up with your bariatric surgeon routinely. During the first couple years following your surgery, you will see your surgeon more frequently. Eventually, you will only need to be seen annually. The annual visits will give you a chance to voice any problems or complaints (like hernias or weight gain). If you've gotten off track, you and your surgeon or other health care provider can discuss what went wrong. This is a good opportunity to get you back on track. If you do fall off the wagon and regain weight, even a significant amount, try to get back on track again with drinking your fluids, eating your protein, taking your vitamins, and exercising. Rededicate yourself to becoming healthy and able to live the life of which you dreamed.

It is also important for you to obtain blood work annually so that your surgeon can check for anemia, vitamin deficiencies, or other problems. Even when you're feeling fine, you can have vitamin or nutrient deficiencies of which you're not aware. It doesn't matter how far out from surgery you are; anemia, vitamin deficiencies, and other problems can occur ANYTIME after surgery.

Another way to keep you motivated to stay on track with your new lifestyle and never go back to being obese again is to become active in the fight against obesity.

The Stigma of Obesity

Obesity is a nationwide problem and is fast becoming a worldwide problem. Two-thirds of the adult population of the United States is overweight or obese. One third of our children are overweight or obese. With obesity come many negative consequences. Obesity is associated with health problems, like diabetes, heart disease, high blood pressure, reflux, and sleep apnea. Associated with it too are the negative ways obese people are treated. As you read on, you may find yourself becoming angry, depressed, frustrated, sad, or tearful. The information presented is not meant to hurt you but rather to educate you. My hope is that by the end of this chapter you will be ready to take action and be an advocate for those with obesity.

Weight stigma—or bias—means that a person has negative weight-related ATTITUDES toward overweight or obese people. These negative attitudes are often displayed by negative stereotypes, for example thinking that obese people are lazy, have no willpower, and have no self-discipline. The negative attitudes are also shown through social rejection and prejudice. Teasing people (like calling someone names), using physical aggression (like hitting someone), and showing relational victimization (like being ignored or avoided) are part of the weight stigma.

Weight discrimination, on the other hand, means that a person SHOWS unequal or unfair treatment toward overweight or obese people because of their weight. This type of behavior can be seen in the workplace, in the health care setting, and in the educational setting.

Opinions that people have about the causes of obesity are part of the reason for the negative stigma attached to it. Some of the opinions included are obesity can be prevented by self-control, patient noncompliance is the reason for failure at weight loss, and obesity is caused by emotional problems. Some people believe that obesity is caused by things a person can control or change—like overeating—versus things that are uncontrollable or irreversible—like genetics.

As the number of people with obesity rises, so does the incidence of weight stigma and discrimination. For whatever reason, it is socially acceptable to have negative attitudes toward overweight and obese people in our society. In fact, it was found in one study of obese people that the rate of weight discrimination was nearly that of race and age discrimination. In women, weight discrimination was more common than racial discrimination. Among all adults, weight discrimination occurred more than discrimination related to ethnicity, sexual orientation, and physical disability. Nearly 60 percent of people in this study also stated that as a result of weight discrimination they experienced at least one occurrence of employment-based discrimination. The study also showed that the chance of being discriminated against seems to go up as a person's weight goes up.

There are several areas in your life where the stigma of obesity and discrimination can come into play: work, health care, and education.

Please remember as you read on that the information addressed may make you upset. Keep pressing on and try to read through this. In order to change attitudes toward overweight and obese people, you need to know what those attitudes are.

Work

When an obese job applicant interviews for a position, the potential employer shows bias by describing the applicant as follows:

- ☹ Lazy
- ☹ Less competent
- ☹ Less ambitious and productive—you can't move as fast, and you fatigue more easily
- ☹ Having poor self-discipline—they believe that all it takes to lose weight is self-discipline, so if you're obese you don't have self-discipline
- ☹ Having low supervisory potential
- ☹ Having poor personal hygiene
- ☹ Being more appropriate for jobs requiring little face-to-face contact

Thin applicants are typically preferred over obese applicants.

Employers show bias toward obese employees when it comes to promotions and career advancement:

- ☹   Prospects for promotion are usually lower compared to non-overweight employees.
- ☹   Managers are less likely to recommend obese employees for promotions.
- ☹   Obese people are less likely to get hired in high-level positions.

Many morbidly obese patients who have come through New Life Weight Loss Surgery Center have been promoted in their jobs AFTER they lost weight—not before.

Employers show bias toward their obese employees when it comes to wages:

- ☹   Obese women earn 12 percent less than thinner females.
- ☹   Obese women are more likely to be in low-paying jobs than thinner women.
- ☹   There are fewer obese men in managerial and professional positions.

- ☹ Obese men are paid less than non-obese men in managerial and professional positions.

Employers show bias toward obese employees when it comes to termination of employment:

- ☹ Obese employees are fired due to prejudiced employers and arbitrary weight standards.
- ☹ Obese employees are fired despite good to excellent records in occupations including teachers, pilots, office managers, state troopers, and city laborers.

Health Care

Hospitals, doctor's offices, and other health care settings can be places of bias. Not only do some health care professionals think and act differently toward overweight and obese patients, but accommodations like seating and blood pressure cuffs that don't fit obese patients demonstrate a lack of respect toward the overweight and obese patients.

Doctors can show bias and discrimination toward overweight and obese patients. Doctors may offer less time, less intervention, and less discussion with obese patients. In fact, in one study it was found that doctors were the second most frequent source of weight stigmatization. Doctors in this study viewed patients as follows:

- ☹ Dishonest
- ☹ Lacking self-control
- ☹ Lazy
- ☹ Noncompliant
- ☹ Unintelligent
- ☹ Unsuccessful
- ☹ Weak-willed

Nurses can show bias and discrimination toward overweight and obese patients too. In the same study, one-third of nurses were reported to admit that they would prefer not to care for obese patients. One quarter of them agreed that obese patients "repulsed them." Just over a tenth of these same nurses preferred not to touch obese patients. Some of the nurses viewed obese patients as follows:

- ☹ Demanding, always needing more help
- ☹ Lazy
- ☹ Noncompliant
- ☹ Overindulgent
- ☹ Unsuccessful

Psychologists in this same study demonstrated their bias too. They were asked to compare average weight patients to obese patients. They described obese patients as follows:

- ☹ Having more health problems

- ☹ Having more severe psychological symptoms
- ☹ Having more negative attributes
- ☹ Having a worse prognosis in treatment

This was only one study, and it does not reflect the views and opinions of every doctor, nurse, and psychologist. It does demonstrate that even in an industry such as health care, bias and discrimination toward overweight and obese patients can and does exist.

Because of the attitudes shown toward obese patients, quality of care may be lacking. Obese patients have been found to be less likely to obtain preventive health services and exams, cancer screening tests, pelvic exams, and mammograms. Obese patients are more likely to cancel or delay their appointments.

Education
Bias and discrimination toward obese children is seen through negative attitudes that can begin as early as preschool. At a young age, obese children are teased and viewed as follows:

- ☹ Having few friends
- ☹ Lazy
- ☹ Mean
- ☹ Stupid

- ☹ Ugly
- ☹ Undesirable playmates
- ☹ Unhappy

This bias continues through high school and college and students are viewed as follows:

- ☹ Excluded from peer activities
- ☹ Lazy
- ☹ Self-indulgent

One-third of overweight girls and one-fourth of overweight boys are teased by their peers at school. Two-thirds of adolescent girls and more than half of adolescent boys report peer victimization (being ignored, being avoided). Teachers view obese students as untidy, more emotional, less likely to succeed at work, and more likely to have family problems. They give obese students poorer evaluations. And physical education teachers criticize athletic abilities of obese students. Obese students are less likely to be accepted to college despite equivalent application rates and academic achievement. Obese students may even be dismissed from college because of their weight.

Depression, anxiety, low self-esteem, poor body image, social rejection by peers, poor quality of interpersonal relationships, potential negative impact on academic outcomes, binge eating, unhealthy weight-control practices—you may already be painfully aware that these can result from bias and discrimination.

But there is hope! Now comes the positive part in all this. You can reduce bias and prejudice toward obese adults and children. How?

Legally, there is not much that can be done. There are no federal laws that exist to prohibit discrimination based on weight. There are roundabout ways to pursue legal alternatives. The Rehabilitation Act of 1973 and the Americans with Disabilities Act of 1990 are two of these alternatives, but they have only been some help. Most cases filed under these categories pertain to weight discrimination in work settings, and only a few cases have been successful. The Americans with Disabilities Act (ADA) questions whether obesity can be called a disability. People who are overweight but not morbidly obese and experience weight discrimination cannot file claims under the ADA because overweight people are not considered disabled. There needs to be legislation created to protect the overweight and obese from discrimination.

Personally, there is more that you can do. First of all, become your own advocate. Think about the situations in which you have been stigmatized because of your weight and decide how to prevent future stigmatization from occurring. Where do you start? Educate others about the physiologic, genetic, and external causes of obesity. Explain to others that obesity is outside of a person's control. Education is a powerful tool. You can reduce or maybe even eliminate the stigma of obesity and prejudice toward obese people by educating others as to the causes of obesity.

The following are causes of obesity:

- ☹ Genetics—this accounts for at least 25 percent (if not up to 75 percent); big people come from big parents and big families; there are two hundred genes that are known to be related to obesity.
- ☹ Metabolism—the lower your metabolism the more fat you store from extra calories; this is beyond a person's control.
- ☹ Overeating—this is part of the cause of obesity; this can happen for many reasons, from emotional to physical; it is not unusual to hear bariatric patients say that before surgery they didn't feel full when they ate; in fact, it's only been since surgery that they know what the sensation of fullness is.
- ☹ Types of fat—fat in and around your belly has a higher metabolic rate than fat around your hips and thighs

⊗   Leptin—protein stored in your fat that sends signals to your brain to tell you to stop eating; with obesity you have much higher amounts of fat and therefore much higher levels of leptin; too much leptin is sending signals to the brain, which then becomes desensitized and no longer listens to the signals to tell you to stop eating.

⊗   Ghrelin—protein produced in the upper part of the stomach that becomes activated when food enters the stomach, telling you to eat until you're full; with surgery, the part of the stomach that produces this is bypassed, and you no longer feel the urge to keep eating.

The following are environmental causes of obesity:

⊗   Automobiles instead of walking or bicycling
⊗   Computer games instead of playing outside
⊗   Elevators instead of stairs
⊗   Escalators instead of stairs
⊗   High-fat foods instead of low-fat, nutrient-rich foods
⊗   High snack consumption
⊗   Larger portions of food at restaurants instead of normal portions
⊗   Low-cost, premade foods lacking nutrients
⊗   Moving sidewalks at the airport
⊗   Riding lawnmowers instead of push mowers

☹   Super-sizing portions at fast-food restaurants

☹   Television

The second thing you can do is find support in other people who are struggling with the stigma of their weight, whether it is family members, friends, coworkers, or other bariatric patients. Be your own support group, educating others about obesity and helping to erase the stigma associated with it. Become a member of The National Association for the Advancement of Fat Acceptance (NAAFA), which is an advocacy group that promotes size acceptance, fights weight discrimination, and publicly campaigns to challenge the stigma associated with being obese.

The American Diabetes Association (ADA) has a Web site you can access with a link to Government Affairs and Advocacy. This Web site addresses diabetes more so than obesity.

Obesity Help has links to the latest stories in the news regarding obesity. This site offers support to patients who are preoperative, postoperative, or who are undecided as to having surgery. This Web site allows you to access public comments on specific insurance carriers in your and other states.

Become a member of Obesity Action Coalition (OAC). The OAC is a nonprofit organization that was formed in 2005. It is dedicated to giving a voice to those affected by obesity. It was formed to build a nationwide coalition of patients to become active advocates and spread the important message of the need for obesity education.

The OAC offers a wide variety of free educational resources on obesity, morbid obesity, and childhood obesity as well as consequences and treatments of obesity. It has a Web site you can access with a link to the Legislative Action Center. This is a great place to start to see the latest advocacy topics, to read about state and federal issues, and is an easy way to contact your elected officials.

Some payers and employers don't recognize morbid obesity as a disease. Therefore, patients are denied access to medically managed weight loss and surgery. The OAC Insurance Guide was created for those wanting to undergo weight loss surgery and provides the tools needed to advocate to your insurer for coverage.

The State Legislation link addresses topics such as lobbying and advocacy. State Guides are available that are state specific and have a more detailed approach to advocating for the obese. You can also obtain Coverage Fact Sheets, which can be used when forming your advocacy initiative to your employer, elected official, or insurance provider.

The OAC addresses state and national issues for adult and childhood obesity including nutrition standards in schools, Medicare rules for weight loss surgery, Medicare-proposed new rules for weight loss surgery, and many newspaper articles published across the country. The OAC issues public policy statements to legislators and insurance providers. The Discrimination link addresses discrimination in the workplace, daycares, public schools, and places of public accommodation. The Federal Government Advocacy link addresses Congress and the White House as well as information regarding increasing funding for research and prevention of obesity.

Patients can be advocates and impact how others view obesity. You can impact decision makers, you can help eliminate negative stigma associated with obesity, and you can demand safer and more effective treatments for obesity.

Don't Hesitate to Speak Out

Be a voice at your place of business. If bias or discrimination is a problem where you work, educate your boss or even the president of your company about the causes of obesity. Educate them on the associated health problems that come with being obese. Educate them on the treatments for obesity, successful (weight loss surgery) and unsuccessful (diets, exercise, diet pills). Educate them on the cost benefit to the company when obese people undergo weight loss surgery—obesity costs the country about $600 billion per year due to the associated health problems and the treatments, medications, doctors' visits, hospitalizations, and days off from work that come with those health problems. When weight is lost, the associated health problems are usually lost too. Many studies have now proven the cost effectiveness of weight loss surgery in the management of obesity-related diseases. A lot less money is spent as a result.

If you know others at work who are obese and want to become healthier, seek them out and help them. Mention times and places for education sessions on weight loss surgery in your area. Start a support group at work and invite people who are obese and people who have had weight loss surgery.

When someone suggests that you've taken the easy way out, first of all, don't blow your top but, second of all, explain to that person how "easy" weight loss surgery has been for you. Describe how "easy" it was to complete mounds of paperwork for your doctors and insurance company. Describe how "easy" it was to get approval by your insurance company for surgery. (If your surgery was covered by Medicare, then it probably was easy to get approval for your surgery.) Describe how "easy" surgery itself was, the anxiety leading up to it and the pain and discomfort after. Describe how "easy" it has been to learn how to eat and drink all over again. Describe how "easy" it has been to motivate yourself to exercise like you should. Maybe once others understand what you actually go through, they won't be so inclined to belittle the process.

When you see your family doctor, cardiologist (heart doctor), pulmonologist (lung doctor), gynecologist or physician assistant, nurse practitioner, nurse, medical assistant, or other health care provider, invite them to attend weight loss-surgery education sessions to learn more about morbid obesity, its causes, and treatments. Many doctors and other health care providers don't believe in weight loss surgery. If they understand that the causes of obesity are not based on character flaws but rather hormone and chemical imbalances in the body as well as environmental influences, they may be more open to supporting weight loss surgery.

Seek out people in your church who are obese and desire a healthier life. Advertise in your church bulletin that help for those who want to undergo weight loss surgery is out there. Offer yourself as a contact person. Mention times and places for education sessions on weight loss surgery in your area. Be a resource for names of surgeons in your area. Start a support group through your church.

Be an advocate within your own family, especially of your children. Go to your principles or school board members and push for healthier lunch options. Request vending machines with sugary pop be replaced with bottles of water. Ask that vending machines filled with chips and sweets be replaced with healthier food choices.

Pregnancy and Having Families

Being overweight or obese can lead to abnormal hormone issues related to reproduction for both men and women. Ovulation and sperm production are affected by abnormal hormone signals and possibly obesity. Gonadotropin releasing hormone (GnRH) triggers the release of luteinizing hormone (LH) and follicle stimulating hormone (FSH), hormones which are critical to the development of eggs and sperm.

Women and Infertility

Many studies have shown that overweight and obese women have more difficulty than normal weight women becoming pregnant. The abnormal secretion of GnRH, LH, and FSH can lead to anovulation (decreased or stopped ovulation). They also have an increased rate of pregnancy loss.

Overproduction of insulin can be associated with morbid obesity. This can lead to irregular ovulation and infertility. This problem can occur with or without having polycystic ovarian syndrome (PCOS). PCOS is associated with overproduction of insulin, obesity, irregular menstrual cycles, anovulation (decreased or stopped ovulation), and increased levels of male hormones. Following bariatric surgery, hormones normalize and fertility improves.

Overweight and obese women have a higher percentage of body fat and, therefore, fat cells. Fat cells produce estrogen. With overweight and obesity, too high an estrogen level results, which negatively influences menstruation and ovulation making it tough to become pregnant. With bariatric surgery and weight loss, estrogen levels stabilize, and menstrual cycles and ovulation can return to normal.

Pregnancy

Pregnancy after bariatric surgery is safe; in fact, it is considered safer than pregnancy while still obese! Women who are obese during pregnancy are considered high risk. If you are morbidly obese during pregnancy, you are more likely to experience gestational diabetes, high blood pressure, a condition known as preeclampsia (high blood pressure, fluid buildup in your body and protein in your urine), fetal distress due to bigger or overly large babies (macrosomia); and you're more likely to require a cesarean section (c-section).

In a study comparing pregnant obese women and women who became pregnant after bariatric surgery, there was a significant difference in the rate of complications. Obese pregnant women experienced gestational diabetes, preeclampsia, and too much weight gain, whereas the women who became pregnant after bariatric surgery did not experience any of these complications. If you choose to become pregnant after bariatric surgery, it is best to wait eighteen months because this is the time after your surgery when you are experiencing rapid weight loss. It is important to wait because it is already difficult enough to meet the nutritional needs for your body. Being pregnant makes meeting your nutritional needs that much more difficult. During the period of rapid weight loss, if you become pregnant, it is possible to deprive your developing baby of needed nutrients. If pregnancy occurs, make sure your obstetrician is aware of the type of bariatric surgery you underwent and how long before your pregnancy the surgery occurred. Expect to be followed by both your bariatric surgeon and your obstetrician throughout and after your pregnancy.

If you underwent the lap band surgery and become pregnant, you will need routine follow-up with your bariatric surgeon because adjusting your band may be necessary. If you are having problems with nausea and vomiting, you will especially need adjustments made to your band. Women who undergo the lap band tend to have less maternal weight gain with no difference seen in the birth weights of their babies. Obstetric complications are minimal including no premature or low birth weight infants.

If you underwent the Roux-en-Y or BPD surgery, you will need to get routine blood tests to watch for nutritional deficiencies during your pregnancy. Women who have undergone gastric bypass have been shown to have lower risk of gestational diabetes, macrosomia (bigger or overly large babies), and C-section. It is very important to be monitored for iron deficiency anemia during your pregnancy.

In women who have had bariatric surgery, breastfeeding following pregnancy is safe. You must be very vigilant about monitoring your nutrition and vitamin supplementation. You also need to make sure you are drinking enough water. Talk to your bariatric surgeon and your obstetrician to make sure your nutritional needs are being met.

Men and Infertility

Overweight and obesity in men can lead to low sperm count and motility problems. Extra layers of fat can surround the testicles and increase the temperature to greater than 96°F. Even a slight temperature increase can cause sperm to die or cause a decrease in sperm production. Hormone irregularities affect stimulation of testicles and can inhibit sperm production. Excess fat causes testosterone to be converted into estrogen, which decreases testicle stimulation. A high body mass index (BMI) correlates with reduced testosterone levels. A high BMI also correlates with abnormal semen analysis with lower volumes of seminal fluid and an increased number of abnormal sperm. With bariatric surgery and weight loss, this improves.

Are Your Children Next?

Remember, big people come from big parents and big families. If both you and your spouse are obese, chances are very good your children will be too. Now that you've had weight loss surgery and you're becoming healthier, help the rest of your family become healthier. No matter how young or old your children are teach them good eating habits. Show by example how to be active. Have them exercise with you. Do things with your kids that involve movement and activity—don't just sit around and watch movies with them or take them out to their favorite restaurant.

Depending on the age of your children, if they are morbidly obese, they may be candidates for weight loss surgery. If they are under the age of eighteen, talk to their pediatrician about surgery. If they are over the age of eighteen, go with them to their primary care doctor and discuss weight loss surgery together. If they decide to have surgery, help them through the process, from completing paperwork and insurance requirements to undergoing preoperative testing (you remember how much fun it was for you?). Guide them after surgery with eating and drinking properly. Exercise together. Succeed together.

There's a light at the end of the tunnel! You're drinking plenty of water and fluids; you're eating right and getting your protein; you're taking all of your vitamins; you're exercising every day; your complications and other problems have been addressed; you're curing the blues; you've got more recipes than you can shake a fork at; your future is looking brighter.

Conclusion

You DID IT! You had your weight loss surgery, and now you have the powerful tool that will help you keep off your extra weight forever. You've changed the way you drink, eat, and exercise. You're working through physical and emotional problems along the way. You're acting as an advocate for yourself, your family, friends, coworkers, and other bariatric patients. It may have taken you awhile to get here, but you made it! Congratulations!

Enjoy your New Life!

Bibliography/Resources

Following are a list of resources used in this book that you may find helpful to access on your own.

Books

Boasten, Michelle. *Weight Loss Surgery: Understanding & Overcoming Morbid Obesity*. FBE Service Network, 2000.

Current Medical Diagnosis & Treatment 2009: 48th Edition. The McGraw-Hill Companies, Inc., 2009.

Current Surgical Diagnosis & Treatment: 12th Edition. The McGraw-Hill Companies, Inc., 2006.

Goldberg, Merle Cantor LCSW, Cowan, Jr, George MD, and Marcus, William MD. *Weight Loss Surgery: Is It Right for You?* Square One Publishers, 2006.

Kurian, Marina S. MD, Thompson, Barbara and Davidson, Brian K. *Weight Loss Surgery for Dummies*. Wiley, John & Sons, Inc., May 2005.

Leach, Susan Maria. *Before and After: Living & Eating Well After Weight Loss Surgery*. HarperCollins Publishers, June 2007.

Pitombo, Cid MD, PhD, TCBC, Jones, Jr., Kenneth B. MD, Higa, Kelvin D. MD, FACS, and Pareja, José Carlos MD, PhD. *Obesity Surgery Principles and Practice*. The McGraw-Hill Companies, Inc., 2008.

Internet Articles

"Cancer Health Center: Gastrointestinal Complications (PDQ®): Constipation." *http://www.webmd.com/cancer/tc/ncicdr0000062736-constipation*

European Society for Human Reproduction & Embryology (2008, July 9). "Obese Men Have Less Semen, More Sperm Abnormalities." Science Daily. Retrieved Feb 11, 2009 from *http://www.sciencedaily.com/releases/2008/07/0807090 84011.htm*

Harvard School of Public Health, 677 Huntington Avenue, Boston, MA 02115, *http://hsph.harvard.edu/nutritionsource*

Hatfield, Heather. "The Quest for Hydration: Drinking fluids is essential to stay alive. But how much do we really need, and what counts in our quest to stay hydrated?" WebMD Feature, *http://www.webmd.com/diet/features/quest-for-hydration*

Huntington Reproductive Center Medical Group. "Reproductive Performance & Endocrine Changes." *http://www.havingbabies.com/infertility-weight.html*

Magee, Elaine MPH, RD. "Why You Need More Fiber: High-fiber foods boost health and help control your weight." WebMD Feature, *http://www.webmd.com/diet/features/why-you-need-more-fiber*

Mann, Denise. "Pregnancy After Bariatric Surgery: Consumer Guide to Bariatric Surgery." Reviewed by Christine Ren, MD, FACS. *http://www.yourbariatricsurgeryguide.com/pregnancy/*

"Obesity Action Coalition: Obesity Stigma." *http://www.obesityaction.org/aboutobesity/obesitystigma/obesitystigma.php*

Puhl, Rebecca PhD. "Understanding the Negative Stigma of Obesity and its Consequences." *http://www.obesityaction.org/magazine/oacnews3/healthqanda2.php*

Puhl, Rebecca PhD. "Weight Discrimination: A Socially Acceptable Injustice." *http://www.obesityaction.org/magazine/oacnews12/obesityanddiscrimination.php*

Schauer Philip R, Schirmer Bruce D, "Chapter 26. The Surgical Management of Obesity" (Chapter). Brunicardi FC, Anderson DK, Billiar TR, Dunn DL, Hunter JG, Matthews JB, Pollock RE, Schwartz SI: *Schwartz's Principles of Surgery, 8th Edition. http://www.accessmedicine.com/content. aspx?aID=809112*

Shared Journey: Your Path to Fertility. "Weight Issues in Infertility." *http://www.sharedjourney.com/health.html*

Sorgen, Carol. "Rev Up Your Metabolism: Follow These 7 Dos and Don'ts to Boost Your Metabolism." WebMD Feature, *http://www.webmd.com/diet/features/rev-up-your-metabolism*

Sparks, Karen MBE, Janeway, Julie M. BBA, MSA, JD, ABD/PhD, and Hendrick, Steven R. MD, FACS. "Infertility and Obesity." *http://www.obesityaction.org/magazine/oacnews7/healthqanda2.php*

The Colon Therapists Network. "The Water Health Report: How eight glasses a day keeps the fat off!" *http://www. colonhealth.net/free_reports/h2oartcl.htm*

"'Thin' Foods to Aid Weight Loss: Do you get plenty of calcium, soy, and fiber in your diet? If not, you're not eating the right "thin" foods." WebMD Feature, *http://www.webmd. com/diet/features/thin-foods-aid-weight loss*

Waehner, Paige. "Exercise for Obese People: Exercising on Your Own: What You Can Do at Home." About.com. Updated December 27, 2006, *http://exercise.about. com/od/weightloss/a/obese_exercise_2.htm*

"Water Retention: What to do about Water Retention." *http://www.bodyandfitness.com/Information/Weightloss/ retention.htm*

Zelman, Kathleen M. MPH. "The Wonders of Water." WebMD Feature, *http://www.webmd.com/diet/guide/wonders- of-water*

Web sites

All Sport drinks, *www.drinkallsport.com*

Allergan Products, *http://www.allergan.com/site* (you can access links to the American Diabetes Association, Obesity Action Coalition and Obesity Help from this site)

American Diabetes Association (ADA), *http://www.diabetes. org/home*

Aquafina, *www.aquafina.com*

Bariatric Choice, *www.bariatricchoice.com*

Bariatric Eating, *www.bariatriceating.com*

Beach Body products, *www.beachbody.com*

Beneprotein® powder, *http://www.nestlenutritionstore. com/bariatric.asp*

Centrum vitamins, *www.centrum.com*

Dasani water, *www.dasani.com*

Doctor's Senior Exercise, *www.doctorsexercise.com*

Flintstones Vitamins, *http://flintstonesvitamins.com*

Fruit$_2$o water, *www.fruit2o.com*

Gatorade drinks, *www.gatorade.com*

Glacéau water, *www.glaceau.com*

Hint water, *www.drinkhint.com*

IsoBreathing® exercise program, *http://www.isobreathing. com/html/isobreathing.html*

Kellogg's Special K products, *www.specialk.com*

New Life Weight Loss Surgery Center, *www.newlifesurgery.com*

Obesity Action Coalition, *http://www.obesityaction. org/home/index.php*

Obesity Help, *www.obesityhelp.com*

Optisource™ high protein drink, *http://www.nestle nutritionstore.com/bariatric.asp*

PowerAde drinks, *www.powerade.com*

Propel Fitness Water, *www.propelfitnesswater.com*

PūR products, *www.purwater.com*

Real Simple recipes, *http://www.realsimple.com/realsimple/ channel/food*

South Beach Diet convenience foods, *http://www. southbeachdiet.com/sbd/publicsite/how-it-works/ convenience-foods.aspx*

Web MD, *www.webmd.com*

Unjury products, *http://www.unjury.com*

Zoic Nutrition Drink, *http://www.zoicbev.com*

Other

Shed and Share Weight Loss Club

- ☺ Participation by anyone is encouraged, including preoperative patients, postoperative patients, family and friends of patients, and anyone wanting to learn more about weight loss surgery
- ☺ Lead by members of the weight loss surgery support team with discussions driven by patients
- ☺ Meets every 2nd Thursday of the month
- ☺ See if you can start a club like this in your area

About the Author

Joanne M. Moff, PA-C, has been a practicing physician assistant for nine years. She received her training at Kettering College of Medical Arts in Kettering, Ohio. She has experience in both general and cardiothoracic surgery, and she recently changed her focus to bariatric surgery. She currently works with Dr. Rita Anderson at Kettering Medical Center.

Okay . . . I've Gone Through Weight loss Surgery; Now What Do I Do?! is truly a labor of love. This book actually evolved from a rather simple idea. During employee orientation at Kettering Medical Center, new hires were encouraged to find ways in which to make a difference in their patients' lives in whatever way they could—big or small. The inspiration to find your "pickle" was introduced. That began the process of seeking out some way to have an effect in bariatric patients' lives. Within the first couple of weeks after starting with Dr. Rita Anderson in bariatric surgery, a "pickle" was discovered. Early recognition of the need for bariatric patients to have support following their surgery was made. In order for the patients to achieve success in the short term with their weight loss as well as in the long term with maintenance of their weight loss and an overall healthier lifestyle, support was seen as necessary. At first, simple ways to offer help were tossed around: a calendar, a mug, or a water bottle with tips, pointers, and reminders on it listing how to live the new lifestyle as a bariatric patient. Then came the idea of a small booklet. The booklet would be interactive, allowing bariatric patients to offer their own helpful hints and suggestions, and there would be input from health care providers as well. As patients gave their contributions, research was being conducted and information was being gathered that would help to explain the whys of the new bariatric lifestyle as well as specific ways to incorporate those lifestyle changes. The booklet grew, going from five sections into eight chapters. It has continued to grow and expand into a full-fledged book covering the most important issues with which a bariatric patient will be faced. The "pickle" that started out as a simple, sweet gherkin has turned into an elaborate, giant dill pickle. What began as a way to help patients in the New Life Weight Loss Surgery Center succeed has turned into a crusade to help all patients who have gone through bariatric surgery succeed. Bariatric patients have seen enough failure in their lives with failed diets and recurrent weight gain. With the support of this book as well as support from family, friends, health care providers, and other bariatric patients, failure will hopefully be a thing of the past.

Book Summary

You have undergone the Lap Band, Roux-en-Y, or Biliopancreatic Diversion with/without Duodenal Switch (BPD). What happens next is up to you. You've been provided with a very powerful tool to help you with your weight loss goals. But how will you make sure you use your tool fully? How can you make sure you are doing what you need to do to maintain your new lifestyle?

To help keep you on track early after surgery as well as years on down the road, it is important to find support in others who have gone through the same thing. That's what this book is all about—offering you support. Some of the information in this book is taken from medical books, journals, and various Web sites. But some of the suggestions are from other patients—patients who have undergone weight loss surgery and know what you are going through. You have an opportunity to read other patients' suggestions and words of advice.

Before your surgery, you were probably told that life afterward would be different, especially with regard to eating and drinking. You were given lots of handouts with information. You went through classes on diet, nutrition, and exercise.

After your surgery, you may start to panic. You have to actually DO what you were taught to do. Suddenly it's not so easy to sip fluids all day long or eat your food slowly. Take a deep breath and relax. Use your handouts and tips from your classes to help you. Use this support book to teach you and guide you in your new lifestyle too. You CAN do this.

Are you wondering if it even matters if you follow all those crazy new ways of eating and drinking? Sure it does. Think of your body as a car. Remember when you got your first car? There was a lot to learn about how to take care of it and keep it working properly. If you didn't take care of your car the way the manufacturer recommended, your car would not run properly, and you wouldn't get two hundred thousand miles out of it. It's the same with your surgery. You need to follow your surgeon's recommendations to "overhaul" your body and improve your "mileage."

As you read this support book, you will find that each chapter tackles a specific problem: drinking enough liquids, eating enough protein, taking the proper vitamins, getting exercise, dealing with depression, finding different meal ideas, dealing with problems and complications, and moving forward after your surgery. You are reminded of the lifestyle changes you need to make. But more than that, the reasons behind the lifestyle changes are explained. And you are given specific examples of how to make those changes real in your life.

Your surgery is the powerful tool you chose to get you started on the road to better health. But like the engine of your car, your tool can only take you so far. It is up to you to keep all the parts of your "car" working properly. This is your new life and your new lifestyle. Your journey toward better health has begun. Let this support book help you continue along the journey, from the first day after your surgery and every day thereafter.

Made in the USA
San Bernardino, CA
23 April 2013